HEALTH
ECONOMICS
AND
DEVELOPMENT

HEALTH ECONOMICS AND DEVELOPMENT

Stuart Wells
Steven Klees

PRAEGER

PRAEGER SPECIAL STUDIES • PRAEGER SCIENTIFIC

Library of Congress Cataloging in Publication Data

Wells, Stuart J   1946-
    Health economics and development.

    Bibliography: p.
    Includes index.
    1. Underdeveloped areas--Medical economics.
2. Underdeveloped areas--Public health.
I. Klees, Steven J., joint author.   II.   Title.
[DNLM: 1.   Economics, Medical. 2. Developing
countries.   W74 W456h]
RA410.5.W45   338.4'7'3621091724   79-24821
ISBN 0-03-055796-8

Stuart Wells is an associate professor at San Jose State University.
Steven Klees is a visiting professor at the University of Natal, Brazil. Funding for research on this book was provided by the U.S.
Agency for International Development to EDUTEL, Inc. The authors
are responsible for its contents.

Published in 1980 by Praeger Publishers
CBS Educational and Professional Publishing
A Division of CBS, Inc.
521 Fifth Avenue, New York, New York 10017 U.S.A.

0123456789   038   987654321

Printed in the United States of America

CONTENTS

LIST OF TABLES

LIST OF FIGURES

HEALTH
ECONOMICS
AND
DEVELOPMENT

1
INTRODUCTION AND OVERVIEW

Our main goal in writing this book is to examine the relationship between health and economic development. Most investigators of health problems in developing countries seem to agree that malnutrition and high rates of disease are related to poverty, but the interpretation of this relationship and the subsequent policy recommendations have led to different analytic approaches. The two main approaches investigated here are disaggregated, sequential policy analysis and structural analysis. The former investigates a sequence of potential policy areas that lead to poor health. If it can be demonstrated that an improvement in health will lead to an increase in economic growth as measured by changes in the per capita gross national product, then it can be assumed that an attempt to influence any factor that can be shown to have a potential effect on health status will also have a positive effect on economic growth. For example, in this book the relationships among health education for the general population, the format of this education, the knowledge and behavioral changes that result, and population health status changes are analyzed. A typical policy recommendation would be to choose that education system that can be demonstrated to have the most positive influence on knowledge, given due consideration to the cost of the alternatives. This cost–effectiveness analysis is considered an appropriate mechanism for choosing among alternatives as long as other, separate analyses have demonstrated that relationships exist between changes in knowledge and health status, and between health status and the economy. The latter relationship allows for conversion from cost-effectiveness to cost-benefit analysis, since benefits are typically measured by economists in monetary terms.

There are many problems with the techniques of microeconomic analysis. The most striking problem is that of ignoring other social institutions that will impinge upon the success of any health education or public health program. These factors include distributions of income, wealth, and power on a national and international scale. When these other factors are examined to determine the potential for success of specific policy recommendations, a structural analysis is adopted in which the context of decisions is considered as important as the decisions themselves. A decision made in one aspect of society tends to be consistent with and constrained by other social institutions.

Despite the problem of ignoring the context of decisions and of other more specific problems related to data measurement and analysis, the tools of microeconomic analysis are increasingly employed by public policy decision makers. Specialization limits the jurisdiction of each decision maker, and thus the context of decisions is frequently overlooked. We emphasize the structural components of decisions because we believe that decisions should be made with a full understanding of the constraints that exist and that an understanding of these constraints may lead to more coordination among social decision makers.

In Chapter 2 we discuss the major health problems experienced within developing countries. This discussion centers on statistics concerning incidence of disease, malnutrition, life expectancy, infant mortálity, health-spending patterns, and availability of medical facilities and personnel. In essence, this type of data provides the framework in which one analyzes and solves health problems regardless of one's particular analytic viewpoint.

Chapter 3 concentrates on specific ways of interfacing the health system with the general population. We discuss some of the main differences between social forces that lead to curative and preventive measures for handling health problems. This is followed by a discussion of different types of health education strategies. The major recipients of health education are health care personnel and the general population: the former are usually involved in formal education systems and the latter in formal or nonformal structures. The chapter concludes with a model describing the relationship of health education to health status.

The structural approach is presented in Chapter 4, in which we discuss the social context of health care from national and international perspectives. From a national perspective we analyze the consistency of the health care structure with the national economic structure. Societies generally seek stability by establishing consistent structures in all social institutions. Additionally, the national economic structure will affect the incidence of disease and other health problems and will provide constraints on possible solutions. The international economic structure also leads to potential problems within countries and provides constraints on solutions. The predominant forms of international economic intervention are world agriculture policies and investment by multinational corporations in developing countries.

The remainder of the book focuses almost entirely on a critical discussion of disaggregated policy approach and microeconomic analysis. Chapter 5 provides a detailed discussion of microeconomic analysis in four specific areas of importance in the delivery of health care or health education: demand, cost, cost-effectiveness, and cost-benefit. Demand analysis provides an understanding of public desire for, and ability to participate in, health care or education systems. Budget constraints often force decision makers to be concerned with cost analysis. In the absence of effectiveness or benefit information, cost analysis uses basic service-level measures and estimates costs of alternative means of providing the service. Cost-effectiveness analysis combines cost analysis with changes in knowledge, behavior, or health status. Cost-benefit analysis translates these health status changes into specific economic changes. For each of the four analytic techniques we describe the basic economic methodology, the types of models used, the items measured, and the problems with the technique.

In Chapter 6 we discuss some of the more important societal issues related to these microeconomic approaches: the relationships among health, education, and economic growth. In these sections we analyze measures and models of national economic growth and the ways in which changes in health status and education can both increase and decrease growth.

In Chapter 7 we consider a specific delivery system for health education and health care: communications technology. We analyze the types of communications technologies and some of their major advantages and disadvantages, and we consider how the usually high initial investment costs affect both the potential social impacts and the methodology described in Chapter 5. We also provide a brief summary of the use of communications technology in health education projects in developing countries.

In Chapter 8 we discuss the basic research methodologies used to answer the questions raised in the microeconomic approach. Specifically, we examine experimental design, econometric techniques, and measurement problems.

Chapter 9 contains a detailed case analysis of a health education project in Tanzania. For the past decade Tanzania's economic policy has stressed self-reliance, decentralization, and development of rural areas. We examine this brief health education project in terms of its consistency with other Tanzanian institutions and policies and in terms of cost, cost-effectiveness, and cost-benefit analysis.

In Chapter 10 we offer a brief summary and concluding remarks.

2
THE HEALTH PROBLEM

Severe health problems exist throughout the developing world although the magnitude of the problems differ—according to a variety of social and economic factors—within different countries. In this chapter we analyze the following: resource availability for health care (in terms of per capita health expenditures); the ratio of physicians and hospital beds to population; longevity, infant mortality, and birthrates; disease incidence; and malnutrition. We conclude with a discussion of the interrelationships among these factors that lead to a magnification of health problems in developing countries.

SPENDING FOR HEALTH

Per capita spending for health is usually significantly lower in developing countries than in developed ones. Jordan (1977) reported that a World Bank survey of 65 developing countries revealed that these countries typically had government-financed health expenditures of 1 percent of gross national product (GNP). Comparable figures for developed countries range anywhere from 4 to 7 percent. The combination of this higher percentage allocation with significantly higher per capita GNP in developed countries leads to extraordinary differences in absolute per capita levels of spending. These differences are illustrated in Table 2.1, which presents the expenditure data reported by the World Bank (1975) for several countries.

In developed countries, the higher health budget (considered as a percentage of GNP per capita) combined with higher GNP per capita has led to higher per capita health spending (for example, $105.16 in the United Kingdom and $180.00 in the United States). On the other hand, per capita health spending in developing countries is considerably lower—for example, $0.80 in Brazil, $3.74 in Bolivia, and

TABLE 2.1

Government Health Expenditures

Country	Health Budget as Percentage of Government Budget	Health Budget as Percentage of GNP	Government Health Expenditure per Capita (in dollars)
Rwanda	8.7	0.8	0.45
Ethiopia	6.9	0.8	0.67
Sri Lanka	8.1	3.6	3.76
Haiti	13.7	0.7	0.78
Kenya	6.4	1.2	0.14
Bolivia	3.6	2.0	3.74
Egypt	8.4	1.8	3.91
Jordan	9.5	2.8	10.10
Turkey	21.4	2.6	8.21
Brazil	1.4	0.2	0.80
Yugoslavia	38.2	10.1	73.75
Venezuela	18.4	4.1	43.18
Soviet Union	5.8	3.4	47.04
United Kingdom	9.5	4.3	105.16
United States	20.0	7.7	180.00

Source: World Bank (1975). Reprinted by permission.

$10.10 in Jordan. As Gish (1970) and Sorkin (1976) pointed out, major increases in the percentage of the budget devoted to health spending in developing countries would do little to close this gap. For example, Sri Lanka has virtually the same percentage of budget allocation for health spending as the Soviet Union but winds up with an absolute spending level of 10 percent less. For equivalent spending, Sri Lanka would have to devote 44 percent of GNP to health spending, an unrealistic figure. In fact, it is reasonable to expect that in the foreseeable future the gap in absolute spending levels will increase. Even if developing countries rapidly increase the percentage of GNP spent on health (at the cost of forgoing alternative government or private spending) and experience a higher GNP growth rate than developed countries, the higher population growth rates in developing countries will result in small changes in per capita health spending. The developed countries with more stable population growth rates and significantly higher GNP per capita will increase health spending more rapidly.

There are three factors that may cause a discrepancy between reported spending and actual spending. The health spending gap is increased between developed and developing countries by the probable differences in private spending. Table 2.1 only reports information on government health expenditures. The large amount of private health spending, particularly in countries with private insurance plans (such as the United States) significantly increases the gap. Differences in income and willingness to allocate income to health expenditures also contribute to this increase.

A second factor is the higher wage structure for physicians and other medical personnel in developed countries, as evidenced by a large migration of physicians to developed countries (World Bank 1975; Sorkin 1976), which leads to an overstatement of the gap for the same input of physician time. However, this inflow of foreign medical graduates from developing countries to countries like the United States results in a subsidization of health training for developed countries and their subsequent need to devote fewer resources to medical training. Hence, health spending by developing countries overstates the resources available to its citizens, because part of that spending is used to train physicians who eventually migrate.

There would be an overall reduction in this gap if it were recognized that much of the health spending in the affluent countries is unnecessary. For example, the United States, with perhaps the highest per capita health spending in the world, ranks fifteenth in infant mortality and twentieth in longevity. These relatively poor statistics may be a result of the distribution of health expenditures within the United States or environmental factors that increase disease incidence. Furthermore, the medical structure in the United States, including government payments, private insurance plans, and physician control of hospitals, creates incentives for excess use of health facilities. Government health plans and prepaid private plans do not create incentives for consumers to control their use of health care facilities since there is no cost attached to facility usage. The consumer has already paid for future visits by paying a fixed amount for all needed care through a private insurance plan or government subsidization. Physicians tend to raise the cost of health care by investing in expensive equipment, knowing that the costs will justify higher rates that will be reimbursed by insurance plans.

RESOURCE AVAILABILITY

The differences in spending patterns may be further seen in the availability of health facilities in different countries. Sorkin (1976)

TABLE 2.2

Physician and Hospital Bed Availability

Country	Population per Physician	Population per Hospital Bed
Rwanda	52,763	771
Ethiopia	73,750	3,124
Tanzania	23,967	625
Kenya	8,914	805
Sri Lanka	3,681	335
Thailand	8,041	972
India	4,399	1,980
China	8,142	1,000
Japan	864	97
Jordan	2,822	706
Egypt	1,516	478
Turkey	2,016	488
Brazil	1,811	282
Bolivia	2,487	561
Venezuela	925	344
Soviet Union	369	86
United Kingdom	756	106
Canada	581	142
United States	616	150

Note: Data are from 1973 except: U.S. physician data are from 1974, U.S. hospital bed data are from 1976, Canadian physician data are from 1976, and Canadian hospital bed data are from 1975.

reported that there were 1.2 million physicians in developed countries and 300,000 physicians in developing countries. Large differences in population between these two regions result in very large differences in population-physician ratios. In fact the United States, with 5 percent of the world's population, has 350,000 physicians (23 percent of the world total).

Table 2.2 gives the ratio of population per physician and per hospital bed in several countries. Comparison of resource availability in Table 2.2 with spending in Table 2.1 shows that spending is not necessarily a good predictor of medical care in terms of the physicians and hospitals available. For example, the Soviet Union has one-fourth the government health spending of the United States and nearly double the availability of physicians and hospital beds. (If private spending were included, the proportion of USSR to U.S. health spending would be even lower.) Similarly, Jordan, which spends only one-tenth as much as the United Kingdom, has one-fourth the physicians and one-sixth the hospital beds on a population basis. This data indicate the higher cost of medical services in the United Kingdom and the United States.

Clearly, though, the data in Table 2.2 are very incomplete, since they fail to suggest the wide range of facilities that are utilized. For example, the cost of training physicians and the small number typically available in most countries have led to the training of para-professionals. Caldwell and Dunlop (1977) reported on the average ratio of paraprofessionals to physicians in 9 Latin American countries and 18 African countries. Dividing these countries into 14 high-income and 13 low-income countries (average GNP per capita of $360 and $105, respectively), they reported that the high-income countries typically had an average paraprofessional-to-physician ratio of 5:1 and low-income countries a ratio of 9:1. Their data show that as income diminishes there is a greater substitution of paraprofessionals for physicians. This fact is consistent with standard economic theory regarding income and demand for goods. As income increases, there is a tendency to increase consumption of luxury goods and to substitute these for goods of lower quality.

NATIONAL HEALTH STATISTICS

The health problems associated with health expenditures and resource availability may be seen in the health statistics typically reported: these include life expectancy, infant mortality, and general mortality. Additionally, data for birthrates and population growth sometimes give an indication of the overall impact of population health status. These five types of data are reported in Table 2.3 for the same countries as reported in Table 2.2.

TABLE 2.3

National Health Statistics

Country	Year of Data	Life[a] Expectancy at Birth	Infant Mortality (under 1 year) per 1,000 Population	Birthrate per 1,000 Population	Death Rate per 1,000 Population	Population Increase (in percent)
Rwanda[b]	1970–75	41.0	132.8	50.0	23.60	2.6
Ethiopia	1970–75	38.1	84.2	49.9	25.80	2.4
Tanzania	1972	44.0	162.5	47.0	20.00	2.7
Kenya	1970–75	48.9	51.4	48.7	16.00	3.3
Sri Lanka	1972	65.8	45.1	29.5	7.70	2.2
Thailand	1970–75	56.1	21.8	43.4	10.80	3.3
India[b]	1973	41.2	12.2	34.6	15.50	1.9
China	1970–75	61.6	55.0	26.9	10.30	1.7
Japan	1973–74	73.7	10.8	18.6	6.50	1.2
Jordan[b]	1970–75	52.3	21.9	47.6	14.70	3.3
Egypt[b]	1974	52.7	100.4	35.5	12.40	2.3
Turkey	1967	53.7	153.0	39.6	14.60	2.5
Brazil[b]	1970–75	59.3	94.0	37.1	8.80	2.8
Bolivia	1970–75	46.8	77.3	44.0	19.10	2.5
Venezuela[b]	1970–75	66.4	46.0	36.1	7.00	2.9
Soviet Union	1973–75	69.0	27.7	18.2	9.30	0.9
United Kingdom[b]	1974	70.8	16.3	13.3	11.90	0.2
Canada	1976	–	–	15.8	7.20	1.0
United States	1976	72.8	–	14.6	8.85	0.7

[a]Average for males and females.
[b]For these countries life expectancy data are from five to ten years earlier than that reported for the other data.

Table 2.3 shows striking differences between developed and developing countries in terms of mortality statistics. Life expectancy at birth in the developing countries is only 60 to 70 percent of that in developed countries. Additionally, infant mortality rates are from 5 to 10 times higher in developing countries than in developed ones. Comparison of data from Tables 2.1, 2.2, and 2.3 fails to show a clear relationship among spending, resource availability, and health statistics. For example, Venezuela has the same infant mortality rate as Sri Lanka but four times the number of physicians and ten times the per capita government health expenditure. Egypt, with twice as many physicians as Jordan and twice the number of hospital beds per capita (but only 40 percent of Jordan's expenditures) has an infant mortality rate five times higher than that of Jordan. India has twice as many physicians and half as many hospital beds as China but a life expectancy only 65 percent that of China and an infant mortality rate more than double.

Birth and death rates for all countries result in major differences in population growth. Whereas death rates in developing countries have been brought closer to the level of developed countries, birthrates remain more than three times as high, contributing significantly to higher population growth in developing countries. Part of the reason for high birthrates is the relatively high infant mortality rate, since people have children knowing that a certain number will die. As infant mortality rates diminish, population growth rates will increase until attitudes change and birthrates begin to diminish. This improvement in both general and infant mortality rates is shown by Sorkin (1976) in a comparison of several developing countries over a 28-year span, from 1943 to 1971. For the eight countries analyzed (Chile, Colombia, Guatemala, Jamaica, Egypt, Mauritius, Thailand, and Singapore) mortality rates in 1971 were one-half to one-fourth of those in 1943. From 25 to 50 percent of the decrease had been accomplished after 1960.

DISEASE INCIDENCE

Although mortality rates have dropped and birthrates remain high, these rates—as Myrdal (1968) pointed out—do not indicate the depth of the health problems faced in developing countries. Debilitating and widespread disease affects great numbers of people and presents a serious block to development in many countries. Wen-Pin Chang (1971) reported on the annual number of cases and deaths attributed to specific diseases throughout the world in the 1960s. There were 150 to 200 million cases of malaria, and death occurred in 1 percent of these cases. There were 15 to 20 million cases of tuberculosis, with 15 percent of the cases resulting in death. Schistosomiasis, a severely debilitating disease, infects 180 to 200 million persons annually. Trachoma, which affects 400 million people, can result in total blindness in 1 percent of the cases and severe vision loss in 14 percent. Wen-Pin Chang (1971) also reported that 500 million people suffered each year from using unsafe water. Caldwell and Dunlop (1977), in their survey of Latin American and African countries, found that clean water was accessible to only 50 percent of the total population in relatively high-income countries and 15 percent in low-income countries. The accessibility rate in rural areas for all countries tended to be one-half the national average. The impact of obtaining water can be seen in the data reported by Blanca and Graham (1974): low income persons in Peru spent 2.7 percent of their income on water, whereas higher income persons spent only 0.7 percent.

The interrelationship of poverty and disease can clearly be seen in the statistics on water usage reported above. Disease is related to poverty in a number of ways. It reduces one's work productivity and earning ability. The lack of income leads to an inability to purchase food and to consequent malnutrition, which further magnifies disease. Additionally, disease reduces an individual's nutrition status as some diseases increase caloric requirements above normal levels and other diseases reduce the body's ability to obtain nutrition from ingested foods.

MALNUTRITION

One of the most serious problems for developing countries is the widespread existence of malnutrition. Wen-Pin Chang (1971) reported that 300 million pre-school-age children suffered from malnutrition. Puffer and Serrano (1971), in a study of selected areas of Latin American countries, reported that malnutrition resulted in 5 to 15 percent of the deaths of children under five and was an associated cause of death in 30 to 60 percent of the cases. Malnutrition problems are increased by differences in calorie and protein requirements, which depend on individual needs. For example, infants require an average of 1,300 calories and 23 grams of protein per day, whereas 3,000 calories and 56 grams of protein are needed by active, growing males. Manual labor in hot climates often requires a sharply increased caloric intake. In addition, pregnant women require 300 more calories and 30 grams more protein per day than nonpregnant women (the normal requirement is 2,000 calories and 46 grams). Lactating females require 500 more calories and 20 grams more protein than the normal level. In the countries they studied, Caldwell and

Dunlop (1977) found an average per person caloric availability of only 2,200; unequal distribution of this amount—which was likely to occur —would cause serious problems for a portion of the populace. Even the average level would create problems for physical laborers or pregnant or lactating women. Schuftan (1977) reported an average daily deficit of 100 to 200 calories in Tanzania.

Malnutrition affects children in several ways: it reduces brain and body size and increases susceptibility to disease. Additionally, malnutrition of pregnant and lactating women results in damage to the fetus. There is some disagreement concerning the link between malnutrition and brain and physical development, owing, in part, to an inability to separate the effect of malnutrition from associated social and economic characteristics. (See, for example, Cravioto, Hambraeus, and Vahlquist [1974] and Lloyd-Still [1976] for a more technical discussion from a medical viewpoint.) Sagan (1977) reported that most brain development takes place from 30 weeks of gestation to 18 months postnatal. Sagan (1977), in an analysis of human intelligence, also discussed a link between nutrition and early brain development, claiming that brain development is negatively affected by protein deficiency. Cravioto (1966) reported that the effects of malnutrition experienced up to the age of six months are not reversible; however, when these effects become manifest after that period, children appear to be able to recover, given a steady nutritious diet. However, Scrimshaw (1967) and Winick and Rosso (1969) reported that the effects of malnutrition before the age of two are not reversible. Kugelmoss, Poull, and Samuel (1964) reported that treatment for malnutrition, especially in early years, resulted in IQ score increases ranging from 10 to 18 percent. Hence, there is controversy over the relationship between malnutrition and brain development and the reversibility of potential negative effects.

Kallen (1969) acknowledged that severe malnutrition was associated with reduced intellectual capacity. However, he felt that lower performance of malnourished children was due to the associated effects of malnutrition, such as lethargy and apathy, and that this limit on a child's performance led to reduced desire to achieve. Since the studies linking malnutrition with development were linked to lower economic status, Kallen asserted that apathy could come from either source. Thus, increasing nutritional standards for low-income children would not necessarily eliminate the other causes of apathy and, hence, would not necessarily increase performance. Moreover, several other studies indicate a relationship between malnutrition and child development (Cravioto and Robles [1965]; Woodruff [1966]; Cravioto and DeLicardie [1968]; Monckeberg [1968]; Stoch and Smythe [1968]). Gopalan (1958) reported that 90 percent of the children of lower socioeconomic status studied in India were in the lower 10 percent of physical size. Jelliffe (1966) also pointed out that malnourished children would be of smaller physical size.

The general conclusion of research into the development of the human brain is that malnutrition leads to a permanent loss in brain development during the period of brain cell division (approximately 30 weeks after conception to 18 months after birth) and that after this period malnutrition reduces brain cell size (not necessarily irreversibly). Therefore, it is clear that malnutrition of pregnant and lactating women leading to malnutrition of the fetus or infant is likely to lead to a situation in which social advancement is difficult, even if all other social factors do not prevent low-income children from moving upward in society.

Belli (1971) made the point that countries would experience substantial economic returns by reducing malnutrition in pregnant mothers and infants. (These economic returns are discussed in Chapter 5.) The nutrition of the mother has been identified as a key problem in a number of studies. The International Conference on Nutrition Education (Kreimer 1977) reported that protein deficiency of pregnant women in Thailand led to below normal birth weights of 2.5 to 2.6 kilograms in low-income families and 3.0 kilograms in higher-income families. Chapra, Gomacho, Devany, and Thomson (1970) also discussed an association between maternal nutrition, birth weights, and infant mortality. Dayton (1969) reported that while more research was needed to determine whether severe or chronic malnutrition of pregnant women was important, the evidence from many studies supported the notion that lactating mothers would need dietary supplements after children reached six months of age.

THE RELATIONSHIP OF NUTRITION AND DISEASE

Perhaps one of the more important impacts of malnutrition is its interaction with disease. Many authors, in discussing this relationship, term the effect synergistic in that malnutrition leads to increased severity of disease and disease leads to increased severity of malnutrition. Sorkin (1976) stated that two-thirds of the 800 million children in developing countries encountered sickness or disabling disease that was brought on or aggravated by malnutrition, specifically, protein-calorie deficiencies. Kallen (1969), Gordon (1969), and Scrimshaw, Taylor, and Gordon (1968) all reported that higher disease incidence, diseases of longer duration, and increased fatality from disease were associated with malnutrition. Additionally, it was stated that disease intensified malnutrition. Scrimshaw (1974) argued that malnutrition led to higher disease incidence by decreasing the person's defense mechanisms and increasing the susceptibility to primary and secondary infections. As pointed out by Gordon (1969) and Kallen (1969), the interaction of diarrhea and malnutrition has created particular problems for young children. Puffer and Serrano (1971) found that in Latin American countries malnutrition was an associated cause in from 40 to 70 percent of deaths due to diarrhea. Appropriate nutrition might have prevented many of these deaths.

Disease aggravates malnutrition by increasing the body's caloric needs. For example, chills associated with malaria can increase caloric requirements to 5,000 calories per day; respiratory tuberculosis, by 20 percent. Dysentery, which renders the body unable to absorb food, increases requirements by 40 percent. Clearly, in situations where caloric deficiencies already exist, the increased need for food will result in an exacerbation of the malnutrition problem. Sorkin (1976) reported that the overall impact of disease was a loss of 20 percent of food ingested but not absorbed.

Malnutrition can also be aggravated by a reduction in agricultural output caused by disease (Malenbaum 1970). Disease has resulted in the loss of large tracts of agricultural land. Hughes and Hunter (1970) reported that a reduction in trypanosomiasis would open lands in East Africa to cattle grazing. Nash (1974) reported that the eradication of malaria in the Rapti Valley of Nepal opened tracts of fertile land for agriculture. This was an especially important effect since the labor needed to cultivate 10 to 12 acres in the valley was the same as that required for two to three acres in the mountains. Hunter (1966) reported that incidents of onchocerciasis, a severely debilitating disease that often leads to blindness, led to emigration from fertile lands in Ghana.

The problems of health in developing countries are severe and complex. Simple resolutions are not possible. As mentioned in this section, many of the serious problems of disease and malnutrition are correlated with socioeconomic status. In addition, agricultural policies and food distribution also lead to malnutrition. All of these areas must be effectively attacked to eliminate health problems. In the next chapter we limit our discussion to different types of specific health interventions.

3
HEALTH INTERVENTIONS

HEALTH CARE STRATEGIES

Curative and preventive health care strategies are the two basic forms of health intervention in a society. Curative strategies are basically those that treat people who have contracted some form of disease or severe malnutrition. Curative practices include most expenditures on hospitals, medical centers, medical equipment, physicians, and paraprofessionals. Preventive measures include inoculation, elimination of environments conducive to parasites, education for better personal health care, and employment of medical personnel and facilities devoted to early disease detection. Typically, these facilities and personnel are the same as those used for curative procedures, and it is unclear if any of the statistics reported below divide hospital or personnel expenditures between the two basic health care methods. What is clear, however, is an overall bias toward expenditures on curative care. As Sorkin (1976) stated, the bias in most countries is toward expensive hospitals and medical personnel concentrated in urban areas, as opposed to low-cost preventive techniques. Alternative explanations for this phenomenon are given in Chapters 4 and 5. In this section we focus upon a variety of statistics that reveal the existence of a relatively large resource allocation toward curative expenditures, with a trend toward increased spending on preventive measures in some countries.

Curative solutions may be much more expensive than preventive ones. Sorkin (1976) reported the following expenditures for curative and preventive approaches to three diseases. Tetanus inoculations cost only $.20, but treatment could cost from $200.00 to $400.00. Drugs to treat tuberculosis and measles are relatively inexpensive at $2.50 and $5.00, respectively; inoculations are even less expensive

TABLE 3.1

Analysis of Government Health Expenditures in Selected Countries

Country	Year	Total Public Expenditures (million dollars)	Percentage for Public Health or Prevention	Percentage for Curative Care	Percentage for Training and Research
Sri Lanka	1957/58	34.3	23.3	74.4	2.3
Tanzania	1970/71	19.5	4.9	80.3	4.4
India	1965/66	236.0	37.0	55.5	7.5
Laos[a]	1971/72	2.3	14.3[b]	19.9[c]	44.8
Kenya	1971	27.8	5.2	83.8	11.0
Thailand[a]	1971/72	83.6	28.1[d]	46.6[c]	19.1
Paraguay[a]	1972	10.0	10.5[e]	84.6[c]	—
Tunisia[a]	1971	15.8	—	86.3[c]	—
El Salvador[a]	1971	30.4	3.3[f]	52.9[c]	1.1
Turkey[a]	1972	303.7	16.3[g]	—	13.5
Colombia	1970	203.0	18.7	79.3	2.0
Mongolia[a]	1972	—	—	—	7.2
Chile	1959	63.8	18.3	77.0	4.0
Panama	1967	28.4	30.0	70.0	70.0
Venezuela	1962	—	18.0	76.5	5.5
Israel[a]	1959/60	82.7	4.9	80.3	4.4

[a]Classification of residual categories of expenditure is unknown.
[b]Expenditure for "environmental health services."
[c]Expenditure for government hospitals only.
[d]Expenditure for "control of communicable diseases, laboratory services, environmental health services and occupational health services."
[e]Expenditure for "campaigns against communicable diseases, maternal and child health and vaccinations and laboratory services."
[f]Expenditure for "immunization and vaccination activities, laboratory services and environmental health services."
[g]Expenditure for "mass campaigns against communicable diseases, immunization and vaccination activities, laboratory services and environmental health services."

Source: World Bank 1975. Reprinted by permission.

TABLE 3.2

Health Budget Expenditures in Tanzania, 1970/71–1976/77
(in percent)

	1970/71	1971/72	1972/73	1973/74	1974/75	1975/76	1976/77
Capital							
Hospital	52	52	27	15	12	22	25
Rural health centers and dispensaries	24	33	35	33	24	34	23
Preventive services	1	2	10	2	8	14	21
Training and manpower	22	13	18	48	55	30	31
Total expenditures (millions of U.S. dollars)	2.76	0.55	1.92	7.25	9.05	9.17	12.22
Recurrent Budget							
Hospital	80	79	72	69	60	60	61
Rural health centers and dispensaries	9	11	18	19	19	20	21
Preventive services	5	4	4	5	12	11	11
Training and manpower	2	3	4	5	6	7	6
Total expenditures (millions of U.S. dollars)	16.97	19.32	24.07	25.71	37.74	42.00	50.74

Note: Percentages may not add up to 100 percent owing to exclusion of smaller expenditure categories.

Source: Caldwell and Dunlop 1977. Reprinted by permission.

19

at $.15 and $.50. While these cost comparisons do not take into account the greater number of people who must receive preventive rather than curative measures, the cost comparison still seems to favor prevention. Moreover, in addition to the treatment cost, one must add the economic loss due to the reduction in work as a consequence of illness. Thus, the benefits of eliminating or reducing disease by preventive measures can be quite substantial.

As Gish (1970) stated, and as is apparent from our discussion of Table 2.1, major increases in percentage of budget expenditures for health care will not result in very large increases to per capita health expenditures. These per capita expenditures will not approach that of the developed countries, the level of which is determined by the choice of an expensive, centralized hospital- and physician-based health strategy. In fact it would seem that opting for a centralized, curative system in developing countries would leave many individuals outside that system. Not only is it unreasonable to expect per capita health care spending of developing countries to approach that of developed countries but it is also not clear that expensive curative health care systems are necessary at all.

Table 3.1 gives data for several countries according to total public expenditures on health, divided among preventive, curative, and training and research programs. The larger allocation for curative expenditures is clear. Most developing countries spend 75 to 85 percent of their budgets on curative measures. However, the trend may be to increase expenditures for preventive measures. Tanzania, which spent 80 percent of its budget on curative measures in 1970/71, has steadily reallocated its expenditures toward more decentralized facilities (rural health centers rather than hospitals) and more spending on preventive measures. These data for Tanzania are reported in Table 3.2 for 1970/71 through 1976/77. In 1970/71, the government spent $2.76 million on capital expenditures and 52 percent of this on hospitals. By 1976/77, the budget had increased to $12.22 million and the percentage of spending on hospitals had decreased to 25 percent (although total spending doubled). A large increase in capital expenditures for preventive measures, from 1 percent of the 1970/71 budget to 21 percent of the 1976/77, was realized. This amounted to nearly a hundredfold increase in total expenditures. Large increases, though not of the same magnitude, were also realized in the recurrent budget.

HEALTH EDUCATION STRATEGIES

Green (1974) distinguished among three basic strategies for health education: individual, community, and professional. A sim-

FIGURE 3.1

An Integrated Health Education System

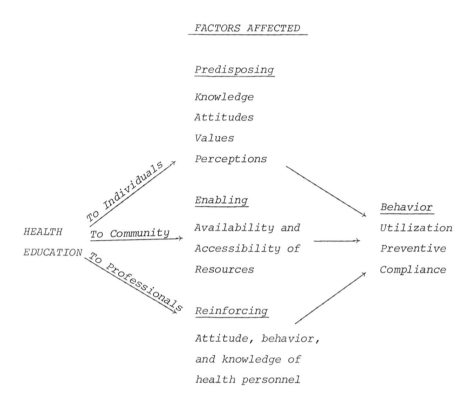

FACTORS AFFECTED

Predisposing

Knowledge

Attitudes

Values

Perceptions

Enabling

Availability and

Accessibility of

Resources

Reinforcing

Attitude, behavior,

and knowledge of

health personnel

HEALTH EDUCATION

To Individuals

To Community

To Professionals

Behavior

Utilization

Preventive

Compliance

Source: Adapted from Green (1970). Reprinted by permission.

plified version of his model is presented in Figure 3.1. Individual
education focuses on predisposing characteristics, which include
knowledge, attitudes, values, and perceptions. Community education
concerns enabling factors: the availability and accessibility of resources. Finally, professional education looks at reinforcing factors:
the attitudes, behavior, and knowledge of health personnel. All three
combine to encourage behavior leading to utilization of health care
facilities, preventive measures, and compliance with health care procedures.

In this model, the entire health care system is seen together
with the education system as an integrated whole leading to curative

and preventive measures. This is an appropriate approach if one believes, as Green does, that the overall goal of health education is to create behavior that leads to changes in health status and eventual social and economic impacts. However, as we have already pointed out, there are other social forces that favor allocations alternative to the curative and preventive elements of the health education system. Therefore, it is reasonable to expect that the entire health education system may be oriented in either direction. For example, Smith (1974) reported that in China the "barefoot" doctor receives a small amount of training (three months of initial training and one to three months each year of continuing education) and has primary responsibility for preventive measures such as health education. Seidel (1972) reported that these personnel received wages one-half the amount normally paid to physicians. However, the training for physicians is much more expensive, and a decision to focus on physician training would likely be tied to a decision to concentrate on curative measures.

Differences in training costs for medical personnel in Tanzania were reported by Sorkin (1976), as follows:

	Pretraining		Training	
Medical officer	6 years	$220	5 years	$3,400
Medical assistant	4 years	220	3 years	500
Rural medical aide	None		3 years	400

Clearly, in a short time and for a fixed budget, one could train many more rural medical aides than medical officers. However, the decision on training must be consistent with the choice between curative and preventive measures.

Djukanovic and Mach (1975) reported on several health care strategies in developing countries (China, Bangladesh, Cuba, India, Tanzania, and Venezuela). These strategies tend to emphasize increased consideration of preventive measures, use of paraprofessionals, health education for the public, and development of decentralized rural health centers. The widespread occurrence of contagious diseases that are transmitted environmentally and whose effects are magnified by poor sanitation conditions has led to emphasis on preventive measures. The success of these measures is dependent on the public's knowledge of nutrition and other health measures, which are in turn supported by an infrastructure of health centers and paraprofessionals.

The decision to allocate resources to either curative or preventive measures is clearly important. While a heavy emphasis on preventive measures seems warranted, strong biases exist for curative systems. The choice of an emphasis for health care cannot be made in the absence of other social development choices. In the case studies of China, Cuba, and Tanzania presented in Djukanovic and Mach (1975) and in the analysis of Tanzania in Chapter 9, it is argued that the path of development is conducive to an allocation of resources to support rural health centers and paraprofessionals. This choice of a development path must accommodate existing social power as physicians in Venezuela resisted the creation of a corps of paraprofessionals in that country. This resistance may have been ill advised. Recently, in the United States, the use of medical assistants has probably led to higher physician salaries by relieving doctors of routine tasks and enabling them to concentrate on more skilled operations.

We turn, in Chapter 4, to a more specific discussion of the national and social structures that affect these resource allocation decisions.

4
THE SOCIAL CONTEXT
OF HEALTH

In the following section we discuss general theories and approaches to the relationship between the economic and social structure of a given country and the health status of its population. For
example, as mentioned in Chapter 3, the decision to concentrate on
a particular type of health care strategy (curative or preventive) is
related to organizational biases favoring either centralized or decentralized systems. In the next section, "Income and Regional Differences in Health Care," we discuss more specific evidence of income
and regional differences in disease and malnutrition incidence and in
access to health facilities. The last section, "The International Social
Structure," returns to an earlier consideration. Throughout our discussion of health problems in the developing world, it was apparent
that many instances of disease and most cases of malnutrition were
associated with lower-income groups. It is clear that middle- and
higher-income people do not typically need to worry about problems
of malnutrition but rather of excess consumption. In fact, the consumption patterns of more affluent people throughout the world are
seen by many authors as a direct cause of malnutrition in developing
countries.

NATIONAL HEALTH STRUCTURES

Poverty is obviously associated with high rates of disease and
malnutrition, but interpretations of causal patterns and proposals for
solutions vary considerably, based as they are on alternative political
and economic theories.

There are two major areas in which one can trace the interaction of the social system with health care: (1) the relationship between the agricultural system and food availability, in which nutrition

levels are directly related to the availability and accessibility of food and (2) the relationship between general economic well-being and health status.

Schuftan (1977) stated that malnutrition is a biological transformation of the socioeconomic, cultural, and historical development of a country. He claimed that his approach was significantly different from the traditional approach, as expressed by Hakim and Solimano (1975), which focuses on policy change within what is seen as a neutral environment. The object of this approach is to improve—usually through education—the nutritional status of individuals and thereby foster economic development. An alternative approach, developed by Jay (1973), Berg (1973), and Schuftan (1978), among others, is to view development patterns as an explanation of nutrition problems. Jay (1973), for example, felt that most malnutrition could be eliminated by concentrating on increasing purchasing power, thus rendering public health programs unnecessary.

Schuftan, Ozerol, and Carter (1977) provided a detailed model of the interrelationship of food production and consumption and the eventual impact on health status and economic development. Simply stated, this model takes the form shown in Figure 4.1. The focal point of the diagram is food consumption, which is a function of the availability of food as determined by food production and distribution and by the accessibility to food as determined by individual socioeco-

FIGURE 4.1

A Simple Food System Model

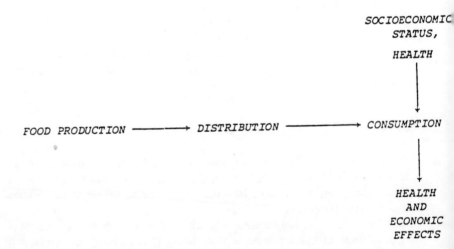

FIGURE 4.2

A Detailed Food System Model

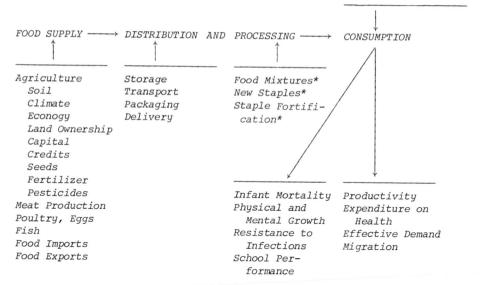

                                                    Income
                                                    Food Prices
                                                    Non-Food Prices
                                                    Habits*
                                                    Family Size*
                                                    Type of Staple*
                                                    General Health*
                                                    Infections &
                                                        Parasites*
                                                    Food Preparation*
                                                    Weaning Practices*
                                                    Sanitation Conditions*

FOOD SUPPLY ⟶ DISTRIBUTION AND PROCESSING ⟶ CONSUMPTION

Agriculture   Storage   Food Mixtures*
   Soil   Transport   New Staples*
   Climate   Packaging   Staple Fortifi-
   Econogy   Delivery   cation*
   Land Ownership
   Capital
   Credits
   Seeds
   Fertilizer
   Pesticides   Infant Mortality   Productivity
Meat Production   Physical and   Expenditure on
Poultry, Eggs   Mental Growth   Health
Fish   Resistance to   Effective Demand
Food Imports   Infections   Migration
Food Exports   School Per-
                                         formance

*Points of intervention of the traditional public health approach to
 malnutrition and disease.

Source: Adapted from Schuftan, Ozerol, and Carter (1977).
Reprinted by permission.

27

nomic status and health. The consumption of food, in turn, affects health and economic status. The more traditional view tends to concentrate mostly on the synergistic effects of health and nutrition and the direct impacts of health on economic status. As Schuftan, Ozerol, and Carter (1977) pointed out, traditional public health programs focus on the individual only in terms of health, education, and habits and ignore the entire food system and other economic influences on food consumption. The wide number of factors affecting nutrition and the small number of items affected by public health programs may be seen explicitly in Figure 4.2.

As is evident from the diagram, the traditional public health approach only affects some factors that have a direct influence on the ability to use food. In part, these factors are related to health status and recognize the synergistic effect that leads to the body's need to consume more food when ill. The other area of concentration is on those factors that can be affected by health education programs aimed at the public. These education programs include those that affect food consumption habits, family size (important in terms of the numbers of individuals among whom the family food supply will be divided), and habits such as food preparation, weaning practices, and sanitation conditions. It should be noted that the public health approach is basically one of preventive care: the education of persons to change a variety of habits to improve nutrition. A more curative approach would treat the health effects of nutrition status. Dayton (1969) expanded the concept of nutrition to include sociocultural effects, such as psychosocial deprivation, but ignored economic effects. The success of this public health approach is severely limited in its application by the income of individuals, prices in the economy, and agricultural and industrial conditions that affect the availability of food.

Recommendations for alternative mechanisms by which public health programs can improve nutrition vary considerably. For example, May and Lemons (1969) suggest four categories of activities to affect malnutrition similar to those in the model:

1. Health education programs to the general public;
2. Health education programs to professionals;
3. Agricultural programs such as quality and quantity of food and harvesting practices; and
4. Industrial programs such as modernization, tax rebates and waivers, and loan programs.

Basically, this approach takes the social structure as given and looks to relatively minor changes within that structure. Schuftan (1977), in his discussion of a more expanded model of the one presented in Figure 4.2, argued that there was a "fundamental bias" to concentrate on characteristics of the malnourished rather than on the characteristics of the social order. While traditional approaches include education and agricultural policies, in general they do not consider a significant alteration in income and wealth distribution, consumption habits of the well-nourished portion of the population, or the approach taken to economic development. Clower, et al. (1976) pointed out that promoting economic development, as measured by growth in GNP, would not necessarily lead to an alteration of living standards for the masses. Harrison (1978) argued that although malnutrition is a result of poverty, a rising GNP would not necessarily be distributed so as to alleviate malnutrition.

While many authors recommend increased availability of credit and education for small farmers, an alternative is to reorganize the landownership pattern away from large, centralized farms to small farms. As discussed in Sorkin (1976) and Ashby, Klees, Pachico, and Wells (1978), research evidence has indicated that crop yields will be higher on small farms. The availability of labor in rural areas also makes this alternative attractive. Bates and Donaldson (1975) pointed out that the research evidence was leading to a shift of international development funds from urban and industrial to rural and agricultural areas. For example, the World Bank has shifted from an average of 8.5 percent of total funds allocated to rural areas in 1948 through 1963 to 20.5 percent in 1969 through 1974. However, Jordan (1977) maintained that many rural development projects focus on a rural elite and ignore the rural class structure. Therefore, for example, a program that improved the health of persons in rural areas would not necessarily lead to increases in productivity, as indicated in Figure 4.2, unless effort was made simultaneously to improve employment prospects.

The model presented in Figure 4.2 is therefore incomplete. There is no inclusion of external social and economic factors that may assist or hinder the conversion of increased health to increased productivity. The main reason is that the model has no reference to aspects of the economy other than those directly connected with agriculture and food distribution. Noticeably absent from this model are the ownership patterns of other sectors of the economy and the structural possibilities that would allow for an individual to improve income as a means of obtaining additional food. It is reasonable to assume that most countries foster social stability by developing consistent social institutions. This consistency is achieved in two major ways: similar organizational structures and cross-support among institutions. If the industrial institutions are centralized with a hierarchical structure one may expect similar structures in the government, medical, and education areas. Also, decisions undertaken in each institutional setting will reinforce those in others. For example,

Galbraith (1967) discussed government support of military expenditures as a means of supporting the technological bias of those in control of large-scale industrial organizations. Gintis (1971) and Bowles and Gintis (1973) criticized education institutions for maintaining social class distinctions. Kleinbach (1974) stated that social stratification extended into, and was reinforced by, medical schools. Jordan (1977) deduced that health efforts would be directed more toward reducing absenteeism of low-skilled employed persons in the industrial sector rather than improving health or even reducing deaths of the unemployed.

Authors who disagree about a variety of political, economic, and philosophical issues would nonetheless acknowledge an overall consistency in a society's institutions. However, the viewpoint that dominates the critical analysis of existing problems of poverty, education, and health throughout the world points to a relatively concentrated private ownership of capital, both nationally and internationally, as the cause of most social ills. Therefore, to understand the prospects for health care in the context of societies dominated by private ownership, one must understand the structure of industry, the primary outlet for private capital. It is important to note that a criticism of private ownership is based on generally acknowledged facts: the distribution of expenditures favoring urban areas and curative systems and the association between poverty and health. The critical interpretation of these facts is that the distribution and association are both based upon, and supported by, private ownership. Therefore, the wide array of programs aimed at specific health problems or incentives to private industry to raise general income levels can only be taken as efforts doomed to failure without widespread effects, since the underlying concentration of economic control is not altered.

Navarro (1975) compared the industrial structure with the health structure in the United States. The industrial structure is highly concentrated with a small minority owning and/or controlling major corporations. He described a hierarchical, pyramidic wage structure with a small percentage receiving high levels of compensation and increasing numbers receiving lower wages. Recent inflation in the United States has tended to serve a widening distribution of income by stabilizing or reducing the real wage (the money wage adjusted for the price level) of many workers and increasing the real wage of management and professionals. This wage structure is repeated in the health sector. Through investment and aid programs to developing countries, this pattern of employment in the health sector in advanced capitalist countries is replicated in the developing world. Additionally, the industrial structure is characterized by large firms with capital-intensive investment. The portion of the economy that is decentralized tends to be labor intensive. This industrial structure is reflected in

medical care in what Jordan (1977) called a bias to in-patient, curative care as manifested in expensive, technology-based hospitals with
expensive medical personnel.

Cosminsky (1977) also provided an excellent example of the impact of biased technology transfer: Western medical practices for
birth deliveries. Traditional techniques in developing countries often
relied on the use of herbs, sweat baths, and a kneeling position. Cosminsky argued that horizontal delivery and the use of forceps are designed to reinforce the hierarchical doctor-patient relationship, the
dependency on related medical technology, the utilization of patent
medicines, and the concept of efficiency in operations in which the
highest value is placed on the doctor's time. Navarro (1977) claimed
that the focus on specialization of medical personnel is a division of
labor similar to that in industry, except that it is more a reflection
of the bias toward treating parts of health problems rather than the
whole. Navarro saw alienation in the medical system as reflected in
placing patients in a state of helplessness and dependency upon physicians.

A more direct relationship to explain the centralization of medical institutions based on consistency and support among institutions
was offered by Rodberg and Stevenson (1977). Capitalism is seen as
a system that requires continuing investment to absorb the surplus
value generated in the industrial sector. Surplus value is the term
applied to profits, seen by many to be a capture of money for no productive work (for example, Schumacher [1973]) or as unearned income
(for example, U.S. Internal Revenue Service). As markets for industrial goods are expanded to their limits, investments are sought
in other areas. Rodberg and Stevenson saw an extension into the tra-
ditionally labor-intensive service sectors, such as medical institutions, as a logical extension of this investment. The subsequent conversion of the service sector into a centralized, capital-intensive sector will naturally follow. They concluded that medical institutions
also absorb surplus labor. In 1969 in the United States, 4 percent of
hospital personnel were physicians; 40 percent were nurses, attendants, and orderlies; and 40 percent were clerical and maintenance
personnel. (The remaining 16 percent of the hospital staff were not
identified.)

Government spending in the health sector may be viewed in a
manner analogous to its support of the industrial structure. For example, Galbraith (1967) wrote that the state supported industry by
supplying trained personnel, underwriting risks and research, and
purchasing products. Navarro (1977) argued that the same trend may
be seen in the health sector wherein state intervention facilitates
capital accumulation by shifting to corporate control of medicine with
a subsidization of technological development and manpower training.

The impact of higher spending and more capital intensity is not structured to improve the health status of the population but to provide an avenue for investment. Eyer and Sterling (1977) argued that the irrelevance of high spending on curative care can be seen in the United States. State welfare programs giving medical access to poorer persons have not brought disease and death rates of poor persons to the levels of wealthy persons, even though access to health care facilities tends to be equal. The point is that the medical welfare programs are used to support the invested capital in medical facilities. Additionally, the potential overspending in many developed countries is supported by research from many sources not founded upon an anticapitalist philosophy. In terms of life expectancy, Cochrane (1972) found no increase with increased health spending in the United Kingdom, Forbes (1967) stated that doubling or halving expenditures would not affect longevity, and Fuchs (1974) stated that the marginal contributions of additional spending were negligible. Yet the bias toward increasing centralization and technocracy in medical systems has been transferred to developing countries. These systems would not be equitable and would conform to a very narrow definition of efficiency: the capability to allocate resources to a demand situation that has been created through control of the structure. Therefore, in developed countries, costs and demands for medical service continue to rise although the effect of the care and the concurrent diseases created by growth of the industrial structure result in small gains in population health status.

One can see a reaction to this trend in several countries, notably Tanzania, Chile (under Allende), China, and Cuba. Many of the changes instituted in these countries have not been solely directed toward health but, rather, have simultaneously attacked health and other social problems related to a social class structure. In Tanzania, according to Schuftan (1977), a series of related reforms have included reduction of income differentials through higher minimum wages, price controls, and a rise in prices of luxury goods; a restructuring of economic institutions including nationalization, a reduction of imports, and an increase in the employment of women; a restructuring of health institutions through an increasing health budget, combined with greater emphasis on preventive measures and rural health centers; a restructuring of political institutions through decentralization and participation; and a restructuring of agricultural institutions through the creation of the ujamaa villages, land redistribution, subsidization of food production, and agricultural credits.

During the Allende years in Chile, changes in several related policies and institutions yielded a 17 percent reduction in malnutrition for children under six. Some of these policies, according to Schuftan (1977), included a milk distribution program, land redistribution to smaller farms, the formation of rural cooperatives, and an attempt to redistribute food resources in a country with sufficient but inequitably distributed food supplies and a foreign exchange food deficit in 1973 of $775 million.

Heller (1973) reported that prior to 1949 China was a disease-ridden country with infant mortality rates of 20 percent. Until 1966 a pyramidic urban-oriented health structure reamined. However, the orientation has changed to an emphasis on rural-based preventive measures, using, in part, traditional treatments such as acupuncture, herbs, and paraprofessionals. The Western model of highly skilled labor combined with a capital-intensive structure results in few individuals willing to work in rural areas. The impact of China's policies can be seen in Table 2.3: for 1970-75, infant mortality had declined to 5.5 percent and was as low or lower than most other developing countries. In Cuba, according to Guttmacher and Danielson (1977), major changes associated with medical care after the 1959 revolution included the nationalization of drug and medical equipment companies, a stress on rural medical clinics with preventive care, and an opening of medical schools to women, blacks, and the working class.

INCOME AND REGIONAL DIFFERENCES
IN HEALTH CARE

The social structure was consciously altered in countries like Chile, Tanzania, China, and Cuba to redress disparities in the allocation of resources according to income and regional differences. This reallocation affected health facilities as well as a wide variety of other resources. In this section we analyze available data that demonstrate the substantial differences within nations in the allocation of health care facilities and disease incidence by income groups and regions.

The differences among income groups can be seen in a variety of ways. Blanca and Graham (1974) reported that the price of clean water was higher for the urban poor in Lima, Peru, and that this accounts, in part, for the fact that they spent 2.7 percent of their income on water while higher income groups spent only 0.7 percent. Oshima (1967), in a study of caloric consumption among income groups in India, reported that lower income groups consumed an average of 1,500 calories per day, middle income groups consumed 2,300 calories per day, and higher income groups consumed 2,900 calories per day.

These differences in access to sanitation and food can lead to situations such as that in Thailand (Kreimer 1977), where birth weights of children from low-income families average 2.5 to 2.6 kilograms and birth weights of children in middle-income families average 3.0 kilograms. North (1970) reported that in the United States respiratory ailments are 10 times more common among children from families of lower economic status than children from families of the highest status.

Paradoxically, a rise in living standards can lead to a decrease in health standards. Reutlinger and Selowsky (1976) pointed out that higher per capita incomes achieved by working mothers could indirectly worsen infant malnutrition, since studies showed a marginal propensity to consume of 5 percent for infant diets, that is, every $1.00 increase in income would result in a $.05 increase in spending on infant diets. However, they estimated that 50 percent of a mother's earnings would be required to substitute for the reduced nutrients from a lack of breast feeding. Thus, some segments of the population suffer from diminishing nutrition despite rising income.

It is not only rising per capita GNP that affects health but also the distribution of that income. Roemer (1977) pointed out that infant mortality was high in countries with relatively high GNP per capita but relatively unequal distributions. This problem was also analyzed in an interesting study of 9 Latin American and 18 African countries conducted by Caldwell and Dunlop (1977). They presented part of their findings for the 27 countries by dividing them into four categories according to average per capita GNP and income distribution as measured by Gini coefficients. A Gini coefficient of 0.0 indicates a completely equal distribution of income: as the coefficient increases, the equality of the income distribution diminishes. The calculation of the Gini coefficient is determined from Lorenz curves as indicated in Figure 4.3. Lorenz curves describe the relationship between the percentage of population and the percentage of total national income received by that proportion of the population. A diagonal indicates the relationship of perfect equality. In this situation, 10 percent of the population receives 10 percent of the income, 25 percent receives 25 percent of the income, and so on.

In Table 4.1, the 27 countries in the Caldwell and Dunlop (1977) study are divided into four categories: those with a high income per capita ($359) and high Gini coefficient (0.574) and three other groups with average incomes per capita and Gini coefficients of $388 and 0.483, $104 and 0.602, and $103 and 0.471, respectively. There are clear differences between the high- and low-income countries according to health inputs: the low income countries spend smaller amounts on health and reach lower health inputs and outputs, as measured by access to water, daily calorie consumption, and infant mortality rates. There are also considerable differences in spending on health care according to income distribution. The countries with the more equal income distribution (lower Gini coefficient) spend an average of 50 percent more on a per capita basis than the other countries. However, the infant mortality rate of the high-income countries with a less equal income distribution tends to be considerably lower.

Similar patterns may be observed in urban-rural disparities. Most of the available data show differences among rural and urban

FIGURE 4.3

Calculation of the Gini Coefficient

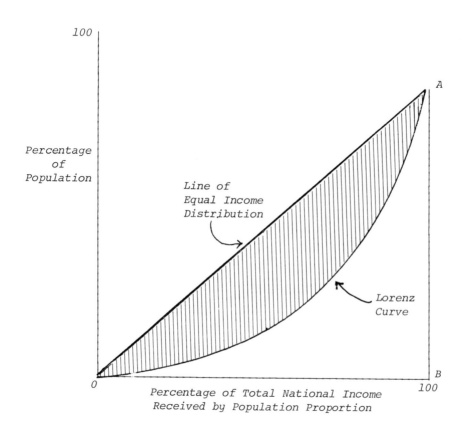

Gini Coefficient = The ratio of the cross-hatched area to the triangular area, OAB.

TABLE 4.1

Measures of Health Status and Resource Commitment in 27 African and Latin American Countries, 1970–73 (countries disaggregated by income concentration and per capita income)

	High-Gini and High-Income Countries (N = 7)	High-Gini and Low-Income Countries (N = 5)	Low-Gini and High-Income Countries (N = 7)	Low-Gini and Low-Income Countries (N = 8)
Average Gini coefficient	0.574	0.602	0.483	0.471
Average per capita income (dollars)	359.00	104.00	388.00	103.00
Average growth rate in income per capita	1.70	2.80	2.30	2.20
Average percentage per capita income spent by government on health expenditures	1.09	0.90	1.67	1.58
Average percentage total access to water	49.30	15.80	48.70	12.50
Average percentage access to water, rural areas	25.50	8.40	27.30	6.50
Average calories per day	2,272	2,091	2,229	2,167
Average support personnel per physician	4.70	8.10	5.40	10.10
Average infant mortality	94.10	143.80	108.70	147.30
Average crude birthrate	44.40	46.80	41.60	47.40
Average crude death rate	14.20	18.90	14.60	20.60
Average population growth	2.91	2.70	2.83	2.64

Source: Caldwell and Dunlop 1977. Reprinted by permission.

TABLE 4.2

Distribution of Medical Doctors between the Capital and the
Remainder of the Country in Selected Countries, 1968

Country	Population per Medical Doctors		
	Nationwide	Capital City	Remainder of Country
Haiti	14,700	1,350	33,300
Kenya	10,999	672	25,600
Thailand	7,000	800	25,000
Senegal	19,100	4,270	44,300
Ghana*	18,000	4,340	41,360
Tunisia	6,486	2,912	10,056
Colombia*	2,220	1,000	6,400
Guatemala	4,860	875	22,600
Iran	3,750	906	6,220
Lebanon	1,470	650	3,000
Jamaica	2,280	840	5,510
Panama	1,850	760	4,400

*Major urban centers instead of capital city.

Source: World Bank (1975). Reprinted by permission.

areas according to access to health facilities. For example, for the
countries reported in Table 4.1, the percentage of persons with access to water in rural areas is half that for the total population. The
difference in distribution of physicians between urban and rural areas
may be seen in Table 4.2. This table provides data for 12 countries
on the ratio of the population to physicians for the country, the capital city (or a major urban center), and the remainder of the country.
On a per population basis, there are about 30 times more physicians
available in the capital cities of Haiti, Kenya, Thailand, and Guatemala than in the remainder of the country. Tanzania, according to
Sorkin (1976), has a similar ratio with a population/physician ratio
of 1,200:1 in the capital and 31,000:1 in the rest of the country.
　　Considerable reallocation between rural and central areas has
taken place in China, Cuba, Chile, and Tanzania, with a heavy emphasis on rural medical units. Gish (1973) pointed out that in Tan-

zania 80 percent of the population is within 10 miles of a rural health center, although most people must walk to the centers. A study of Tanzania by Van Etten (1972) found—as one would expect—that utilization of hospital facilities diminished as people came greater distances to the facility. For example, at one hospital 50 percent of the outpatients came from within 10 miles, 20 percent from 10 to 20 miles, and the remainder distributed from areas further removed from the hospital. The shift in resources in Tanzania from hospitals to rural health centers may be seen in Table 3.2. Recurrent budget expenditures increased from 9 percent of a $16.97 million budget in 1970/71 to 21 percent of a $50.74 million budget in 1976/77, a tenfold increase in absolute expenditures. This shift in expenses is justified according to a cost/capacity analysis undertaken by Sorkin (1976), examining equivalent capital and recurrent expenditures on one regional hospital or 15 rural health centers. The regional hospital would have a capacity of 9,000 inpatient admissions and 400,000 outpatient visits and would cover a population of 10,000 to 30,000. The 15 rural health centers would have a capacity of 15,000 inpatient admissions and 1,000,000 outpatient visits and would cover a population of 30,000 to 500,000.

The reallocation of medical expenditures in Tanzania is also indicated in data analyzed by Caldwell and Dunlop (1977). Even though capital and recurrent expenditures for hospitals increased between 1972 and 1976, the increasing population resulted in an increase in the population covered per hospital. In the same period of time, however, the population per health care facility declined owing to the increase in the number of rural health centers.

Interestingly, although rural areas typically have far lower access to health facilities, their health status can be higher. For example, in the Bangladesh case study reported in Kreimer (1977), the average daily caloric consumption in rural areas was only 2,251, but consumption in urban areas was even lower—1,732 calories. These differences are related to the potentially easier access to food in rural areas. Food access, in general, is a major problem for developing countries and, according to many authors, it is dependent upon world agricultural systems and multinational corporations. These relationships are discussed in the next section.

THE INTERNATIONAL SOCIAL STRUCTURE

Tudge (1977) claimed that sufficient food would be available on a worldwide basis if farmers grew crops for nutrition rather than profit and if they avoided single, cash crop agriculture. He further argued for a greater emphasis on small farmers, a minimum use of technology, and a reduction of waste in developed countries. Many authors, such as Lappé and Collins (1977), reason that the emphasis on food scarcity is a myth and that sufficient food is available if managed and distributed more equitably. Reutlinger and Selowsky (1976) calculated that the worldwide caloric deficit is 419 billion calories and that this is equivalent to 38 million metric tons of grain or 4 percent of world production. In a later study, Harrison (1978) estimated that the world production of 1.3 billion metric tons of grain would provide 3,000 calories and 65 grams of protein daily—equivalent to the nutrition standards for a physically active 170-pound male—for each of the four billion people in the world.

The four major interrelated factors mentioned most frequently as influencing food deficits in developing countries are food consumption patterns in developed countries, agricultural practices in developing and developed countries, the oil crisis, and the effects of multinational corporations. Food consumption patterns in developed countries have been termed "excessive." The excess is represented not only by overconsumption but also by heavy consumption of beef protein. For example, Lappé (1975a) stated that 16 pounds of grain are required to produce one pound of beef. In fact, the United States, though a major beef producer, is the leading importer of beef in the world. Berg (1973) pointed out that during the 1960s, meat production increased in Central America but meat consumption declined. In Costa Rica meat production had increased by 92 percent, but per capita consumption had declined by 25 percent. Most of this meat wound up in U.S. franchise restaurants.

The impact of beef protein consumption can be seen in other ways. According to Borgstrom (1974), for example, American livestock consume six grams of grain protein for every gram of meat protein created. Patton (1968) claimed that 50 percent of total acreage in the United States was directed toward food for livestock consumption. Much of the grain fed to livestock is high in protein and nutritionally sufficient for protein consumption of humans. Lappé (1975b) discussed the protein content of three groups of grain and the amount fed to livestock. For example, soybean contains 35 to 40 percent protein by weight, and over 90 percent of the crop is fed to livestock. Corn, barley, and oats have protein contents ranging from 8 to 14 percent, and 90 percent of this crop is fed to livestock. Although only 24 percent of the wheat crop is fed to livestock, it is also a good source of protein, containing 11 to 14 percent. Additionally, feedlots in the United States rely on heavy protein ingestion to increase fat—which, though basically nonnutritious and potentially harmful, improves the taste of beef.

Overconsumption is not confined to the United States; it occurs in all developed countries. In fact, the developed world imports more protein from the developing world than it exports to it (Borgstrom, 1974). Europe imports one-third of the African peanut crop (an excellent protein source) to feed its livestock. Holland, a known dairy-producing country, is a leading importer of milk. Lappé (1975a) stated that the average person in the United States eats twice the daily protein requirement. Since protein is a daily need and cannot be stored by the body, any amount consumed in excess of the daily requirement is converted to carbohydrates for energy. There are more efficient ways to provide carbohydrates, notably through grains. U.S. livestock can be reduced by 25 percent, according to Lappé (1975a) and still provide enough protein from beef to meet each person's daily requirements.

The impact of this beef consumption on agricultural land can easily be seen. As stated previously, 50 percent of agricultural land in the United States is used to feed livestock. More important, there is only one acre of culturable land per person in the world, whereas 3.5 acres are needed to sustain one meat diet (Lappé 1975a). Food problems in developing countries may be increased by agricultural practices in developed countries in more ways than illustrated above. Analyzing U.S. agriculture, Lappé (1975a) stated that since 1940 large productivity increases have created a food surplus "problem." It is difficult, if not impossible, to sell the excess at a profit. The food is not going to developing countries because of their lack of foreign exchange and escalating food prices. Brown and Eckholm (1974) reported that wheat prices had tripled from 1972 to 1973 and that, in a 24-month period, soybean prices had quadrupled. The inability to purchase food and the excess supplies have led to a situation that Lappé (1975a) described as an institutionalization of waste in agricultural and nutrition practices. In 1972 this led U.S. farmers to withhold one acre from planting for every 4.5 acres harvested. In that year $3.6 billion was spent to subsidize nonplanting, an expenditure equivalent to three times the food aid bill to developing countries. As Lappé succinctly observed:

> Since our economic system does not recognize need,
> but only "effective demand" (an economist's euphemism
> for ability to pay), we have been totally unable to recog-
> nize waste.

While agricultural and food practices in the developed countries have reduced the world food supply, there have been other international economic forces that have also had deleterious effects on developing countries. One of these factors has been the dramatically increased price of oil in international markets. In the developed world the impact has been inflation, which has perhaps resulted in a curtailment of leisure-time activities. In the developing countries the impact has been starvation. In the United States, according to Brown and Eckholm (1974), 75 percent of energy used in agriculture is for transportation, processing, and preserving food. The remainder, presumably, is absorbed in fertilizer production. Fertilizer is a major component of agriculture, and over 50 percent of nitrogen fertilizer used is processed with natural gas. The additional productivity of fertilizer would be higher in the developing world. With similar soil conditions, rice yields in Bangladesh are one-third those in Japan. Similarly, India produces half the agricultural output of the United States, although both countries have equivalent amounts of cropland. There is clearly potential for greatly increased productivity in India. The price of energy has risen at the same time that the U.S. dollar—the major reserve currency held by developing countries— has been severely devaluated. The Green Revolution in developing countries included the use of fertilizer. Hence, developing countries have agricultural systems dependent on fertilizer and are increasingly unable to obtain it.

The lower yield on agricultural lands is accompanied by a heavy pressure from economic and political forces to devote agricultural lands to cash crops. The economic theory used to promote these policies is that cash crops lead to the accumulation of foreign exchange, which the country can use to buy industrial goods and food to compensate for the lost agricultural land. This theory is based on the principle of comparative economic advantage, which basically leads to allocation of resources in each country allocating resources to those products that it can produce relatively more efficiently than other countries. In the developing countries, this process led to the planting of a series of crops with no nutritional value: sugar, tobacco, coffee, tea, cocoa, and rubber. This agricultural decision was made for the developing countries when they were colonized and large tracts of land were grouped in plantations. However, while the theory partially worked in terms of accumulation of foreign reserves, there was no internal process that caused the recipients of agricultural profits to forgo luxury goods in order to purchase food for the population.

According to Revelle (1974), coffee has become a primary means of economic subsistence for 14 countries, subjecting the entire economies of these countries to price fluctuations of a single commodity. The international economic pressures that lead to reallocation of agricultural land previously used to grow nutrition crops can be seen in the case of Brazil, where a hectare planted in carnations has a value of 1 million pesos while the value of land planted in corn or wheat is only 7,500 pesos (Barnet and Muller 1974a).

A major impetus for many cash crops stems from multinational corporations, which control much of the supply. However, this is only one of the harmful impacts attributed to multinationals (Barnet and Muller, 1974b). Another major impact of these companies has been the heavy advertising in developing countries for nonnutritious products, such as Coca-Cola and white bread. This advertising has stressed status, convenience, and, in the case of substituting for mother's milk, modernization, and has led in many instances to the neglect of nutritious foods.

In this section we have analyzed a wide variety of national and international political and economic problems that have exacerbated the health problems confronting developing countries. From the model in Figure 4.2 and the discussion in this chapter, it should be apparent that one must separate the two main health problems in developing countries, namely, disease and malnutrition. Public health policies aimed at preventive measures for eradication of contagious diseases have some possibility of success if changes required in lifestyles do not involve major expenditures. While biases exist toward curative techniques in many social structures, there is little benefit derived from avoiding public health programs. However, when any public health program requires major expenditure, public or private, its chance of success diminishes. Public expenditures for health must compete with alternative programs. These decisions are typically made by a more centralized urban-based elite, whereas the health expenditures are needed in the rural areas in addition to urban slum areas.

Public health programs directed toward eradicating malnutrition have less likelihood of success. These programs must compete with far less controllable international forces that reduce the amount of nutritive food available and advertise for personal expenditures on nonnutritive foods.

To many, the appropriate policy is to alter the major social forces that relate to health problems. However, among others who see major change as unlikely or undesirable, there is a search for analytical tools that aid in sensible choice among a set of more limited alternatives. Thus, many policy analysts have been attracted to the microeconomic tools of demand, cost, cost-effectiveness, and cost-benefit analysis, which are believed to help one to choose among alternative policies that differ marginally, and retain the status quo in terms of distribution of power. These methodologies for economic analysis are discussed in the next chapter.

5
MICROECONOMIC ANALYSIS OF HEALTH DECISIONS

BASIC PRINCIPLES OF MICROECONOMICS

> If economists can help to rationalize and make more explicit the decision-making process . . . they will be making their own contribution to health and the economy.
>
> Fuchs 1972

> Planning should be based on more than humanitarian principles.
>
> Sorkin 1976

> Planning should be based on more than humane principles. It can cost a nation significant amounts of money to alleviate malnutrition. There also can be a significant opportunity cost of making these expenditures in light of other possible expenditures for equally worthy programs.
>
> Cesario, Simon, and Kinne 1970

> While informed judgement is useful and important, excessive use of its defeats the principal purpose of model building which presumably is to replace judgement with an objective evaluation.
>
> Cesario, Simon, and Kinne 1970

Microeconomics is based upon allegedly rational, objective, quantifiable criteria for choosing among alternative investments, both private and public. The application of microeconomic analysis to health problems is not a new topic (see, for example, Weisbrod 1961; Crystal and Brewster 1966; Rice 1966; Smith 1968). Because society's resources are scarce, any allocation of a resource to some specific investment removes the possible use of that resource from alternative investments. In the public sector, resources may be allocated to a wide range of projects including agriculture, education, health, housing, and conservation of environment. These same resources may have been used in the private sector for a wide range of goods and services. Hence, there is an opportunity cost associated with any resource allocation decision. Opportunity cost is a valuation of that resource in alternative activities. Economists make this valuation based upon certain explicit assumptions: individuals act in their own rational, economic self-interest; individual decisions are independent of each other; market power is not exerted in the economy; and all individuals have access, at no expense, to information regarding prices, qualities, and production technologies for goods and services. If all of these conditions hold, the prices assigned to goods and services in the economy can be viewed as reflecting the value that society as a whole places on the goods. The first assumption above is based on an economic interpretation of human behavior and perhaps of human "nature." It is this characteristic that leads to a preference for private ownership in the economy and, perhaps as well, to the occurrence of overconsumption of food and the production of nonnutritional cash crops in the face of worldwide malnutrition and disease. While this assumption—of economically self-interested behavior exemplified by profit-maximizing producers and utility-maximizing consumers—may or may not hold, the other assumptions of the perfectly competitive market are rarely borne out.

There are many situations in which the decisions of individuals affect others. For example, the decision of some people to purchase a good leads to a production process that may cause pollution of the environment of others. The persons in the polluted environment will then need to allocate resources to clean-up activities or to medical care to reverse the negative effects of pollution. What economists call an "externality" occurs whenever one allocation of resources in response to supply and demand conditions results in the imposition of a resource allocation decision on others. It should be noted that most economists do not consider an externality to occur when one group of consumers desires a product, such as coffee or tobacco, and prime farmland is allocated to meet this demand, thus relegating food production to less fertile land where there is a greater resource need to produce the crop. This use of land for cash crops rather than food crops is seen as an efficient allocation of resources, since the underlying economic theory does not question the distribution of wealth, which directs consumer demand.

The assumption that there is an absence of market power is also not realistic. Clearly, there are large corporations that can greatly influence market prices as well as affect demand through mass advertising. The increase in oil prices that created havoc for agriculture in developing countries was not a result of a free interplay of market supply and demand. The price increase was mostly the result of power politics among a few producers. Large corporations with market control are a fact of life in developed countries. In fact, the extension of these corporations to multinational operations has had a wide variety of impacts. Although we have mentioned some of the negative impacts reported in the literature, other authors, such as Thompson (1975), have discussed the benefits derived from this concentration of economic power. A wide range of products, lower prices, and technological progress are among the more important benefits mentioned.

Finally, there is considerable controversy over whether information is available. The fact that many persons in developing countries allocate their income from needed nutritious foods to nutritionally useless foods, such as soda and coffee, is seen by many critics to be a direct result of the market power exerted through advertising. They feel that the "information" contained in advertising does not focus on the inherent functional characteristics of the product but reinforces product decisions based upon irrelevant criteria, such as product packaging, brand name, and status for food products. Supporters of the "free" market system (that is, free from government interference that restricts the scope of business decisions) claim that advertising merely informs consumers of the availability of products, and continuing sales of any product is based upon quality and satisfaction of consumer desires rather than any psychological forces of advertising.

Economic analysis based on these free market assumptions is often considered to be an objective approach to decision making. No individual's values dominate; rather, the convergence of values of many people determines resource allocations within a society. Within this structure, resource allocations may be based on or result in unequal resource distributions, but these inequalities are usually considered outside the scope of such economic analyses of efficiency. Thus, in the remainder of this section we pass over these equity issues and concentrate, instead, on some of the techniques—including demand, cost, cost-effectiveness, and cost-benefit analyses—used to aid in decision making.

Demand analysis can be used to estimate the market's desire for different types and amounts of medical care service, including health education programs, hospitals, smaller health care facilities, and physicians. Cost, cost-effectiveness, and cost-benefit analyses are three means economists use to evaluate the impact of supplying medical service to meet demand. The cost element of the analysis is the same for all three. The difference is the type of impact assessed relative to the cost of the program.

In cost analysis one usually compares an alternative's cost with the level of service provided, such as number of students reached, number of hospital inpatients, number of outpatients serviced, or number and type of a variety of specific medical services rendered. In cost-effectiveness analysis one translates these service levels into health status variables, such as mortality and morbidity statistics, for segments of the population. In assessing a health education program, one often measures knowledge or attitude change as a result of the intervention, but this is an intermediate output toward health status. Finally, in cost-benefit analysis, changes in health status are converted to monetarily measurable impacts—specifically, changes in productivity. Though such changes are related to economic growth and changes in GNP, we reserve a discussion of this topic for Chapter 6. In our discussion in this chapter of cost-benefit analysis, we concentrate only on improvements in productivity for an average individual receiving the health education or service.

In the remaining four sections of this chapter we discuss methodologies, models, examples, and problems for each of the analytic techniques.

DEMAND ANALYSIS

Demand analysis is used to assess the desire of the public for a certain level of medical service or health education. While many commentators on health problems discuss concepts of "need" in terms of societal health problems that should be corrected, economists focus on demand, or the willingness of people to pay for a service. A good or service will only be supplied by a competitive economy if there is "effective" demand. Effective demand may be interpreted as the payment for services that is sufficient to induce private producers to provide the service at a profit. Therefore, since economists consider income distribution as given or as a separable issue, the analysis of any services to be supplied is based more on ability to pay than on actual social need. (This is true even when governments provide the "demand" for a service.)

The estimate of a demand for a service is basically a price-quantity relationship, as shown in Figure 5.1. For any of the demand curves depicted (these are assumed to be linear), demand decreases as the price of the service increases, and vice versa. For demand curve A, a decrease in price from P_1 to P_2 will be accompanied by an increase in demand from Q_1 to Q_2. The position of the demand curve is affected by a variety of factors, including income,

FIGURE 5.1

Demand Curve Relationships

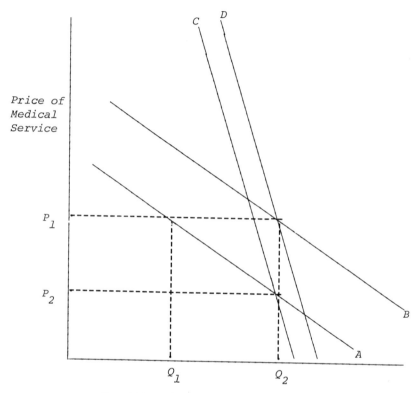

Quantity of Medical Service Demanded

prices of other goods, preferences, and education. Any given demand curve such as A or B in Figure 5.1 is estimated for a given set of income, prices, preferences, and education. If any of these factors change, the demand curve will shift to a different position. For example, an increase in income could result in a shift in demand from curve A to curve B and an increase in demand from Q_1 to Q_2 at price P_1. Government policies of subsidization of medical services will cause movements along a specific curve (for example, P_1Q_1 to P_2Q_2 on curve A). Public health programs, by changing attitude or education, will cause a shift in demand curves (for example, from curve A to curve B).

Ruchlin and Rogers (1973) suggested that medical services are different from other goods and services in that medical insurance or government subsidization may decrease the amount that individuals pay. This may result in demand curves such as C and D, in which demand is relatively insensitive to price.

It is important to note that demand curves, as depicted in Figure 5.1, are usually drawn for a specific period of time and represent the aggregate market demand. Therefore, shifts in market demand curves are affected by general social changes in preferences, income, and the production of other goods and services. Differences among individuals in terms of income or preferences are accounted for in the individual demand curves that are used to construct a market demand curve.

A typical economist version of demand analysis was undertaken by Rosenthal (1974). In his analysis, he attempted to estimate the demand for hospital beds as affected by price, income, insurance, and a variety of factors assumed to affect preferences, such as age, marital status, sex, race, urbanization, education, and population per dwelling. In the econometric technique of linear regression analysis (described in more detail in Chapter 8) one can allegedly determine a demand curve (the quantity-price relationship), since the impacts of factors affecting shifts in demand (income, insurance, and preferences) are statistically controlled.

Equations of the type estimated by Rosenthal (1974) are attempts to provide specific quantification of general process models of consumer behavior. An example of a process model to describe demand is presented in Figure 5.2. In this model the factors that change the likelihood of taking preventive health actions are analyzed. In economists' terms, this is an effective demand. The demand for preventive care is influenced by a variety of items affecting preference or perceived threat of disease: perceived susceptibility and seriousness of the disease, socioeconomic status (age, sex, race, income, and so on), sociopsychological factors (personality, peer and reference group pressure, and so on), structural variables (knowledge about the disease, prior contact with the disease, and so on), and cues to action (mass media campaigns, advice, illness of family member or friend, newspaper or magazine articles, and so on). All of these factors affect a person's perception regarding the threat of disease, the benefits of taking preventive action, and the barriers to preventive action (including cost of preventive care). The difference between benefits and barriers affects the likelihood of taking action. One can see from this model the potential impact of health education interventions through mass media campaigns and knowledge about disease.

The perceived benefits and barriers to action are associated with the two purposes for which a good or service may be used,

FIGURE 5.2

Demand Model for Preventive Care

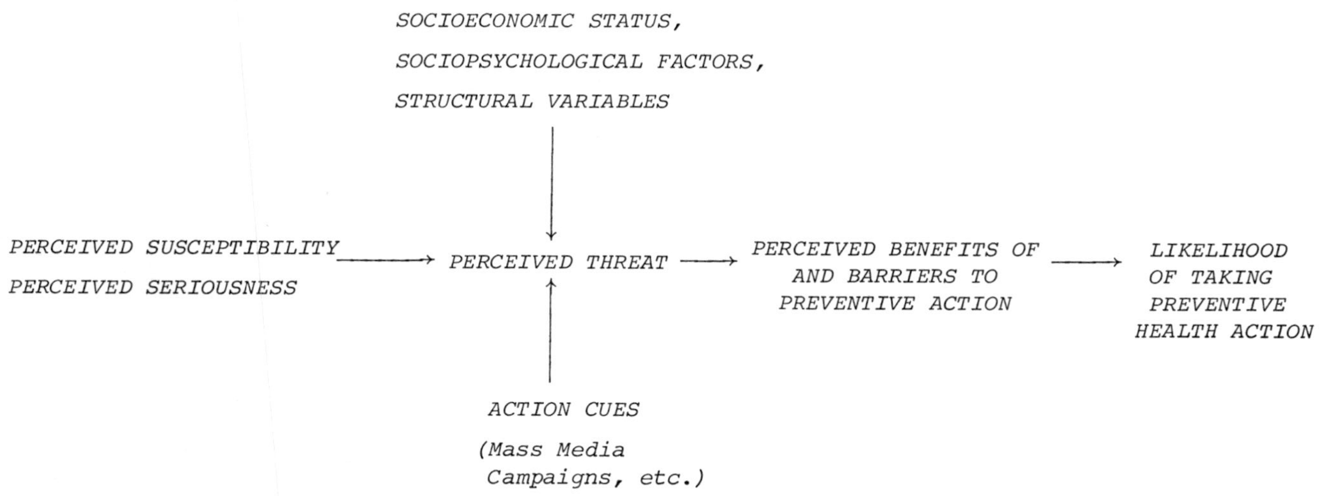

namely, consumption and investment. Mushkin (1962) and Grossman (1972) analyzed medical care in terms of consumption and investment components. Consumption components are associated with the satisfaction one gains from being healthy or protected from disease. This type of satisfaction is similar to that attached to the use of any goods, such as automobiles, furniture, and clothing. The investment component of the good is the one more subject to economic analysis, since the benefits of the good are accrued through economic returns such as increased income. In order to calculate a derived demand for health services, Chernichovsky (1977) analyzed expected lifetime earnings as a sum of the discounted values of the wage for each year adjusted by the probability of surviving and the probability of being physically capable of working. (The concept of "discounted values" is explained in the section that follows.) Chernichovsky used the following equation:

$$LE = \sum_{i=1}^{n} \frac{P^s_i P^c_i W_i}{(1 + r)^i} \qquad (5.1)$$

where LE = the discounted sum of lifetime earnings, P^s = the probability of surviving in year i, P^c = the probability of being physically capable of working (given that the individual has survived) in year i, W_i = the expected wages in year i, and r = an interest rate used to discount future earnings.

Other equations could be estimated to relate the change in probabilities of survival and work capability with the demand for health services. In a similar vein, Becker (1965) assumed that the major resource that households had to allocate was time of household members. This time allocation resulted in a given labor supply. Based on this principle, Florencis and Evenson (unpublished) analyzed the allocation of nutrition to household members. They felt that nutrition would go to the highest wage earners (the adult males) in the household if nutrition were viewed as an investment good.

In analyzing the relationship between income and demand for any food, Johnston and Millar (1960) calculated an income elasticity (the percentage increase in spending for a 1 percent increase in income) for all foods in developing countries equal to 0.6. Mellor and Lele (1972) estimated the marginal propensity to consume (the percentage of a one-unit income increase) of different income groups in India. Lower-income groups had a marginal propensity to consume all foods of 0.76 (76 percent of any additional income would be spent on food), whereas those with income ten times higher spent only 34 percent of additional income for food. Moreover, the type of food consumed by different income groups was affected by price as much as nutrition. For example, lower-income groups spent 55 percent of their incomes on grains, food of lower cost, and moderate nutrition; higher income groups, only 2 percent, with a heavier dietary reliance on higher-cost, more nutritious food.

Although most of the analyses above are concerned with effective demand as a means for analyzing the market for health services, it is not necessarily the best approach for national development. The cycle of poverty is evident in that lower-income families must choose which members of the family can receive appropriate nutrition and must spend large percentages of income on food: little then remains for other health services. In these situations those with a greater ability to pay can bid health services away from lower-income groups, thus leaving them with little or no health care. Hall (1974) discussed needs assessment models for predicting the requirements for health care personnel as an alternative to the economist's effective demand approach discussed above. His biologic demand model assesses the health problems expected to exist in a country; his service target model determines the level of service to be made available. Both models depend on heavy governmental involvement in the health sector in order to respond to such conceptions of social need.

COST ANALYSIS

Within the microeconomics framework we are discussing, the existence of a consumer demand for a service is not sufficient to justify its provision. This demand must be balanced with the cost of providing the service. In analyzing the costs of a health care system, economists often measure the value of resources used to produce a given level of service. To measure the output of the model, Cohen (1967) used a weighted index of several service level measurements, including patient days, X-ray procedures, laboratory tests, outpatient visits, and operations. Leslie (1978a) discussed audience size as a measure of the "outreach" or service level of health education programs. The major problem with level-of-service measurements is that little or no consideration is given to the quality or impact of services. Therefore, service levels should be viewed simply as a guide to discussions of cost. In the remainder of this section, we will discuss some basic concepts of cost analysis (see Klees and Wells [1978] for a more detailed discussion) and apply them to health systems.

The prime consideration of economic analysis is the allocation of scarce resources. Thus, in analyzing any health system it is necessary to list explicitly all resources used in the system, including personnel, facilities, and equipment. In view of the fact that health care systems are often operated for several years, one should list the resource requirements according to year of operation. Resources should be listed in physical terms, so that one knows the number and type of specific resources according to the general categories. In order to project resource requirements, it is necessary to predict service levels and determine the amount of resources to be assigned to meet that level of service. For example, the service target method for predicting health personnel needs discussed by Hall (1974) involves decisions regarding the number of people to be served, the types of services to be made available, and the number of physicians or other personnel needed for the service.

Once a listing of resources has been completed, it is necessary to apply cost figures to each, since economists determine the total value of personnel, equipment, and so forth by assigning a price to each. This leads to two possible evaluation methods: opportunity cost and market price. In measuring opportunity cost, the attempt is made to assess the social value of resources in alternative investments. Therefore, if volunteers are used in a medical system, one must assign a value to these persons. Similarly, a value should be assigned to donated physical resources. Additionally, one must assign a value to the time the patients spent using the health care facility or participating in the health education program. However, since it is difficult to assess social value as expressed through alternative resource use, it is common to use market prices, which are supposed to reflect the opportunity cost of resources in a perfectly competitive economy. One uses the wages earned by persons of equivalent capability or in their normal work activities to calculate a value for volunteer and patient time. A major structural problem with this model is that decision makers in the public or private sector often consider only the market prices of those resources that must be paid for from the budgets within their own control. The first item normally excluded from any analysis in this fashion is time of patients. This leads to models of medical care "efficiency" that focus only on the higher-paid physicians and the use of medical facilities.

When the public sector decision makers ignore costs incurred by patients or other participants and the value of their time, misallocations of resources can occur. It is possible that the costs to the individual will be sufficiently high to prevent use of the system, or, in the case of health education, to make compliance with the suggested health practices impossible. Decision makers who formulate health education programs typically consider only budget expenditures used to produce and distribute the program; the costs to participants of changing their diet, altering community sanitation, or utilizing health care facilities are often ignored.

In a previous section we reported on the costs of health care in Tanzania over a period of seven years. In this table there was a division of government budget expenditures in terms of capital and recurrent expenses. (Expenses incurred by patients were not included.) Capital expenses are used for resources that have a serviceable life greater than one year; recurrent expenses are used for resources that will be used within a one-year period. Personnel expenses are considered recurrent expenses, since the services of individuals are utilized during the year and must be paid annually. In order to compare costs of different systems with different amounts of capital and recurrent expenses fully, it is necessary to place these costs on a similar basis. To do this an annual value is calculated for capital expenses by multiplying the expenditures by an annualization factor, $a(r,n)$, given by the following equation:

$$a(r,n) = \frac{r(1+r)^n}{(1+r)^n - 1} \qquad (5.2)$$

where r is an interest rate, and n is the number of years for which the equipment or facility can be used. If the interest rate is equal to zero, the annualization factor becomes $1/n$ and is equivalent to dividing the cost of the resource by its useful life (for example, a $100 piece of equipment lasting five years would have an annual value of $20). A positive interest rate will increase the annual value of the capital equipment. There is controversy over the appropriate interest rate to use (see Feldstein 1964; Marglin 1967), but a reasonable approach is to use the average real rate of return in the economy (the rate of growth of the economy adjusted for inflation). The justification for using any interest rate at all is that it will represent the opportunity cost of committing financial capital to a particular project and forgoing alternative investments. Using an annualization factor, one can obtain an estimate of the total cost (the monetary value of all resources) of an entire health care system or portions of it. One would add the recurrent costs in a particular year to the annualized value of facilities and equipment available for use.

One other concept used in many reports of system costs is average cost. Average cost is simply total cost divided by some specific direct output of interest, such as number of patients or number of students. Most reports of costs of medical systems do not contain significantly more detail than annual budgets for capital and recurrent costs or an average cost figure for treatment. We discuss some of these reports below. It is important to note that an average cost figure helps to place alternative decisions on a more comparable basis. Total cost figures do not indicate the relative capacity of systems. Therefore, it is possible that the more expensive system serves fewer patients.

One other important cost methodology that will be useful in comparing costs is the discounted value method. This technique is especially useful in choosing between alternatives in terms of cost-effectiveness and cost-benefit analysis. The main reason for using a discounted value method is that costs (or effects or benefits) may be realized in different years. For example, preventive treatment costs are incurred in the present, curative treatment costs in the future. Suppose that, for a given population over a five-year period, one has a choice between two systems. Preventive treatment might cost $1 million during the first year only, for example, 1980; assuming 100 percent coverage, there would be no curative costs incurred in future years. This preventive system might require inoculation of the entire population or a health education program that created an immediate change (an unlikely occurrence) in a specific health practice. Suppose the alternative is a curative treatment system that is expected to cost $275,000 per year for years 2, 3, 4, and 5 (that is, 1981, 1982, 1983, and 1984). If one simply added costs, the curative system would have a total cost over a four-year period of $1 million, and the less-expensive preventive system would be chosen. However, simply adding costs from different years of the project does not give one an accurate picture of the total since one has not accounted for the opportunity cost of invested capital. This opportunity cost is incorporated into the analysis by realizing that it is preferable to delay expenditures to the future because such expenditures have a lower value than expenditures in the present. To calculate the discounted value of the stream of expenditures for a specific project, one multiplies each expenditure by a present value factor, $PV(r,n)$, given by:

$$PV(r,n) = \frac{1}{(1 + r)^{n - k}} \qquad (5.3)$$

where r is an interest rate, n is the year of the project, and k is the initial year of the project; and then sums the total of the discounted value, DV, as follows:

$$DV = \sum_{i = k}^{n} \frac{C_i}{(1 + r)^{i - k}} \quad \text{or} \quad \sum_{i = k}^{n} PV_i C_i \qquad (5.4)$$

where C_i is the cost in year i.

It should be noted that in using the discounted value method, the costs in any year of the project, C_i, include the total commitment to expenditures in that year. Capital expenses are not annualized but, rather, included at full value in the year in which the equipment or facility is first used. This does not cause any calculation problem, since in the first cost-analysis technique one annualized capital costs using the lifetime of the resource. In the discounted value method, one assigns a value to a capital resource in the initial purchase year and each replacement year. Thus, for example, equipment with a five-year life will be purchased in years 1, 6, 11, and so on. The methods are essentially equivalent.

In our simple preventive versus curative treatment example above, the discounted value of preventive treatment would remain at the original $1 million, since it is expended in the initial year. However, the discounted value of the expenditures on the curative system would become $975,000, assuming an interest rate of 5 percent, and would be preferable (on a cost basis only) to the preventive system. It should be noted that this cost comparison does not include an important indirect cost of treatment: the productivity loss due to absenteeism, inefficiency, and disability (Cesario, Simon, and Kinne 1970). The productivity issue is discussed in greater detail below.

In the remainder of this section, we discuss reported costs for various health-related systems and the implications of these costs. In viewing treatment of malnutrition, Bengoa (1970) reported that one-half million persons in 37 developing countries were hospitalized in 1968 for an average of 90 days at $7.50 per day.' Berg (1973), using similar cost figures, stated that there were 10 million children in these countries who would require hospitalization at a total annual cost of $7 billion. Three items should be noted in the reporting of this data. First, the analysis views only hospital treatment costs and not other economic losses due to malnutrition. Second, comparable figures for preventive treatment (basically the assurance of a nutritionally adequate diet) are not calculated. Since the hospital and diet expenses would be incurred each year, one could simply calculate the total number of persons who could receive supplements to bring their diets to adequate nutritional levels for an annual expense of $7 billion. Finally, the manner in which the cost of $7.50 per day is calculated is important. Perhaps the most appropriate procedure would be to sum the recurrent costs of the facility (personnel and basic supplies) with the annualized value of capital expenses (the facility and all equipment) and divide by the capacity of the facility (the number of beds multiplied by 365). This calculation would give a part of the daily cost per inpatient. If the hospital does not operate at capacity, total cost should be divided by expected utilization level. To either of these average figures one should add the costs that specifically vary with each patient, such as drugs, food, and laundry.

As mentioned previously (see "Health Care Strategies" in Chapter 3), Sorkin (1976) reported the following preventive and curative costs (in dollars) for inoculation against three diseases:

Preventive		Curative	
Tetanus	0.20	200–400 (treatment)	
Tuberculosis	0.15	2.50 (drugs only)	
Measles	0.50	5.00 (drugs only)	

Both cost reports are incomplete in that the inoculation costs do not include facility expenses, and treatment other than drugs for tuberculosis and measles is excluded. While curative procedures appear significantly more expensive than preventive procedures, it is necessary to realize that curative procedures are applied only to those who contract the disease, whereas preventive measures need to be applied to large segments of the population. It is difficult, if not impossible, to know which persons will become ill and require preventive treatment. Therefore, the average cost comparison used by Sorkin (1976) in this instance is not appropriate. One should use the discounted value method and compare total costs for each system of health care for an entire segment of a population.

Of additional importance to the choice of preventive and curative measures is the potential for economies of scale in preventive measures. If one considered the entire set of diseases to which a particular population might be subject, it might be possible to construct health campaigns or education programs, such as that in Tanzania (see Chapter 9), that emphasized preventive measures for a large number of those diseases. Alternatively, it would be possible to institute an inoculation program that simultaneously included several diseases. The economies of scale of these preventive measures derive from the ability to use the same facilities, equipment, and personnel to fight several diseases simultaneously.

As an example of a comparison of treatment costs, Bodenheimer (1969) compared a mobile health unit with ten stationary health posts. A mobile health unit would have an initial capital cost of $4,500 and an annual recurrent cost of $25,000. A single health post would have an initial capital cost of $10,000 and an annual recurrent cost of $6,000. Considering the lifetime of capital equipment, Bodenheimer calculated that ten health posts would be three times as expensive as one mobile unit but have four times the utilization. This is an example of an instance in which average cost analysis is useful.

The need to consider effectiveness measures is evident in several cost analyses. For example, Sorkin's (1976) comparative cost analysis of medical care training in Tanzania indicated the following:

	Pretraining	Training
Medical officer	6 years at $220 per year	5 years at $3,400 per year

| Medical assistant | 4 years at $220 per year | 3 years at $500 per year |
| Rural medical aide | None | 3 years at $400 per year |

It is apparent that on a simple cost basis one could train far more rural medical aides than medical officers for the same expenditure in a shorter period of time. With more aides available, more persons could be served. However, without any knowledge of health status changes, it is not possible to choose among the types of medical training.

Similarly, Sorkin's (1976) comparison of one regional hospital with 15 rural health centers showed inpatient utilization 1.7 times higher and outpatient utilization 2.5 times higher for the rural health centers. Capital and recurrent costs were the same for both alternatives; thus, assuming the same lifetime for capital expenses in both systems, the average cost per patient (inpatient, outpatient, or a weighted average of the two) would be lower for the rural health centers. On a cost basis alone, one would choose the rural health centers. However, without knowing the effects of the treatments, it is not possible to choose.

The same average cost problem for different health care facilities is evident in Segall (1972). His data are reported in Table 5.1. Though the pattern of average costs is apparent, the effects of the different treatments are not clear.

TABLE 5.1

Health Facility Treatment Costs
(in dollars)

Type of Facility	Cost of Treatment per Case	
	Tanzania	Kenya
National hospitals	77.20	54.40
Regional hospitals	33.80	25.00
District hospitals	25.30	12.35
Health centers	0.73	0.58
Dispensaries	0.33	0.30

Source: Segall 1972. Reprinted by permission.

COST-EFFECTIVENESS ANALYSIS

The calculation of costs provides an important and necessary component of the criteria economists use to choose among alternative investments. However, costs alone are not sufficient. An estimate of the effectiveness or benefits of the programs must be made. Leslie (1978a) gives four measures of health status: mortality, morbidity, anthropometry (size and weight measurements), and biochemical test analysis. Statistics indicating nutritional standards in terms of protein, calories, and vitamins are also important. The most readily available statistics are mortality and morbidity for an entire population. However, it is more important to obtain these statistics and the nutrition level on a disaggregated basis according to demographic variables such as age, sex, region of country, and income. A disaggregation helps to indicate where programs need to be directed.

Effectiveness of education systems can be analyzed in two stages: the first is the one frequently analyzed by educators—knowledge and attitude change; the second focuses on changes in behavior and associated health status resulting from knowledge or attitude change. Measurements of knowledge and attitude are perhaps most easily obtained by testing program participants. However, a program that appears cost-effective from the viewpoint of knowledge change does not necessarily result in signficant behavioral changes.

There are two ways to view the impact of such an education program. On the one hand, it may be claimed that the program was not successful and was not cost-effective inasmuch as few or no behavior changes resulted; on the other, it may be argued that knowledge change is one aspect of the social system, that there are many other social factors that affect behavior, and therefore, that education is not sufficient for solving this particular problem. From this perspective it is impossible to judge the efficiency of the education program without considering aspects of the social system that might promote or deter the behavior desired. For example, an education program may be very successful in transmitting knowledge regarding nutrition, but, if no resources are available to allow changes in nutrition, there will be no change in health status.

As an example of this disaggregated policy approach, one may consider the Reutlinger and Selowsky (1976) analysis of the cost-effectiveness of four alternative programs to induce changes in nutrition levels: (1) a general food price subsidy, (2) a food price subsidy for specific foods, (3) a food stamp program, and (4) an income transfer. Cost-effectiveness was based upon the program cost to increase nutritive diets. On this basis they felt that alternative 3 would be the most cost-effective, since food stamps could only be used by a given group of people for specified foods. The other three alternatives were not specific enough and were dependent upon the income and price elasticities for nutritious food of the target population. Income and price elasticities (the percentage change in amount demanded percent change in income or price), which economists use to summarize demand relationships, are important since each of the programs results in a reduction in price or an increase in income for the target groups. These price or income changes induce people to buy more nutritive foods to different extents (depending upon individual income and price elasticities). The program that gives the greatest effect for a given cost—food stamps according to this study—is considered the most cost-effective.

One problem with all these alternatives is that there is no analysis of any concurrent education program that, through the teaching of nutrition, could change the population's food preferences. All the programs change either amount of income or price of food. Price and income elasticities determine new consumption patterns for food and are affected by attitudes or knowledge that can be changed by health education. The cost-effectiveness of a program combining health education with one of the Reutlinger and Selowsky suggestions may thus be higher than that of either program implemented independently.

In an analysis of 96 experiments in family planning, Cuca and Pierce (1978) reported that fertility rate was used as the dependent variable in many instances. However, in many cases a proxy variable measuring knowledge, attitudes, or acceptance was used. It is clear that unless these direct program impacts are translated into behavioral changes (as measured by a fertility rate) the program will not achieve its goals. In a manner similar to Reutlinger and Selowsky (1976), they also analyzed the effects of economic incentive programs not related to education programs, including incentive payments for using birth control, deferred payments based on the number of births or time without pregnancy, and payment for "voluntary" sterilization. A cost-effectiveness measure might aim at lowering birthrates relative to the costs of the resources used by the program. However, as Cuca and Pierce mentioned, all the programs raise ethical questions, and the cost-effectiveness question may be the least important criterion for choosing such a program.

In an analysis of cost-effectiveness, Klarman, Francis, and Rosenthal (1968) calculated the costs of a variety of treatments for chronic renal disease in terms of the costs of the program and life expectancy of the patient. The basic costs in treatment are a onetime kidney transplant (with a repeat operation in the case of failures) or a continuing program of blood transfusion and drugs. While the quality of life is better for the transplant patients, the analysis is based only on cost differences between the two methods. Because the transplant method is basically a onetime expense and the other is a continuing expense, it was necessary to compare the cost-effectiveness of the alternatives using the discounted value method.

The technique Klarman, et. al., used for cost-effectiveness analysis is a common one: hold the effectiveness levels of the alternatives constant and compare the relative costs of each, choosing the alternative that is least expensive. This type of choice, as viewed by economists, is illustrated in Figure 5.3. For simplicity it is assumed that each alternative uses the same two inputs (for example, personnel and equipment), but in different combinations, to produce the same output levels. Curve O in the diagram is an isoquant, the locus of different input combinations for a given output level. Curves B_1 and B_2 are alternative fixed-budget levels. They are drawn as straight lines to indicate fixed prices for the inputs regardless of the amount

FIGURE 5.3

Cost-Effectiveness Analysis for Fixed-Effectiveness Level

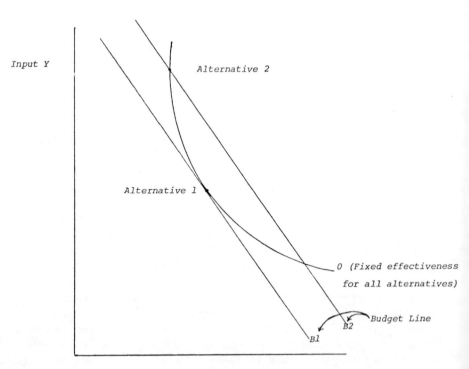

FIGURE 5.4

Cost-Effectiveness Analysis for Fixed Budget

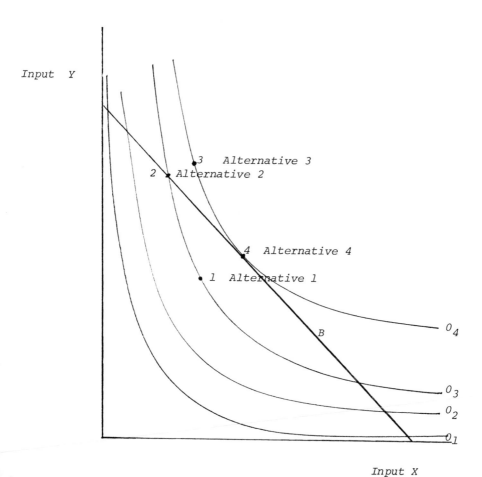

purchased. The isoquant is curved to represent the economist's belief in diminishing marginal productivity of inputs; that is, as more of a given input is used, holding other inputs constant, the contribution to additional output decreases. Alternatives 1 and 2 are both in the set of feasible, efficient alternatives that yield a fixed-output level (for example, a given patient life expectancy, as in Klarman, et al. [1968]). Alternative 1 is chosen because it is the least expensive. This is illustrated by placing it on the lowest possible budget line to achieve the effectiveness level specified.

An alternative cost-effectiveness approach is represented in Figure 5.4. In this instance the alternative that reaches the highest effectiveness level for a given budget is chosen. Economists think of this situation in terms of an infinite combination of different input and output levels, represented by an infinite number of isoquants, with O_1 through O_4 illustrating just a few. The most cost-effective decision, assuming that one spends a fixed budget B, is to buy that combination of resources that gives the highest output, represented by the highest possible isoquant—output O_4, alternative 4. Alternative 1 (or any point under budget line B) uses less than the budget allocated and thus produces less output. Alternative 2 uses up the budget but gives less output than alternative 4 (producing O_3 instead of O_4). Finally, alternative 3, although it too produces output O_4, is not feasible since it requires more than the fixed budget (as does any input combination above the budget line B).

It is frequently the case, however, that practical political propositions for alternative systems are assumed to have different costs as well as different effects. That is, instead of the economic choice model above which assumes that there are an infinite number of input combinations for producing any possible output, in reality only a limited number of alternatives are considered. Under these circumstances, a decision maker might think that the alternative with the lowest cost-effectiveness ratio should be chosen. For example, suppose alternative A decreases infant mortality 20 percent at a cost of $1 million and alternative B decreases mortality 10 percent at a cost of $300,000. It is clear that alternative B has a more favorable cost-effectiveness ratio ($30,000/percent decrease versus $50,000/ percent decrease). However, if alternative B is not repeatable—that is, if the program cannot be implemented twice to receive a decrease of 20 percent for $600,000—it is not clear that one would not prefer to have a greater decrease in infant mortality, even though the cost for the second 10 percent decrease is more than double that for the first 10 percent. Once this situation arises, cost-effectiveness no longer offers a clear selection criterion.

An additional problem occurs in cost-effectiveness analysis when there is more than one effectiveness measure. In all of the analyses above, a single measure was implied. Once a program can affect more than one relevant output measure, as is usually the case, one needs a means of indexing the measures to derive a quantitative criterion for choosing among the alternatives. The index would be some weighted average of the relevant outputs, wherein the weights would be subjectively determined by the decision makers. Since determining and agreeing upon such weights are difficult, economists favor cost-benefit analysis, in which one attempts to convert the health status changes to economic changes, as measured by the theoretical objectivity of the price system.

COST-BENEFIT ANALYSIS

Most economists argue that any evaluation is incomplete if an attempt is not made to examine resources used and outcomes attained in terms of their monetary value. (For a contrary view, see Duckham, Jones, and Roberts [1976]. They suggested using energy to measure inputs and outputs in the food cycle, since energy has a longer-lasting value than money.) Economic theory argues that cost, effectiveness, or cost-effectiveness analyses alone provide only very limited information needed for societal decisions among alternatives.

If costs and benefits can be expressed in monetary terms, economists then use several alternative summary quantitative measures to depict the benefit-cost value of each alternative. Three measures are most common, all based on the discounted value method of summarizing money values over time (as explained above). The first method is to use a constant interest rate and choose that alternative with the highest ratio of discounted benefits to discounted costs as given by:

$$\text{Benefit-cost ratio} = \frac{\sum\limits_{i=k}^{n} \dfrac{B_i}{(1+r)^{i-k}}}{\sum\limits_{i=k}^{n} \dfrac{C_i}{(1+r)^{i-k}}} = \frac{\sum\limits_{i=k}^{n} PV_i B_i}{\sum\limits_{i=k}^{n} PV_i C_i} \qquad (5.5)$$

where B_i is the benefit in year i and C_i is the cost in year i. Second, one can subtract the present value of the costs from the present value of the benefits (that is, the numerator minus the denominator in equation 5.4) to yield the net present value of each alternative. Third, one can use an internal rate-of-return analysis by setting the benefit-cost ratio in equation 5.4 equal to one and solving for the interest rate, r. In that case, one chooses the alternative with the highest rate of return.

Although all three may yield slightly different results under different circumstances (see Cohn 1976), in all cases one is trying to allocate scarce resources, indexed according to market prices, to produce the highest economic returns. The predominant economic benefit postulated to result from health programs occurs via improved job performance through higher productivity on the job or fewer days lost to disease. (Reduced curative medical expenses are also an important consideration.) The validity of cost-benefit analysis is based on an important premise of competitive markets: persons are paid a wage equivalent to the value of their marginal product. This premise is based on all the assumptions of competitive markets, in general, and most specifically depends on the employer's profit motivation. Profit-maximizing producers will continue to hire workers until the wage paid to the last employee is equated with the additional output that employee contributes, multiplied by the price of that output. If wages are determined in competitive markets, the wages paid to employees of similar capabilities will be equal. In this situation, economists examine the earnings of persons with different health levels, or directly examine the productivity of these persons multiplied by the output market prices, in order to determine the economic benefits of health programs.

If one used only this cost-benefit approach for health decision-making criteria, one would likely derive optimal levels of malnutrition or disease incidence. These "optimal" levels would be the point at which the rate of return of further programs to reduce malnutrition would be less than the return that could be earned elsewhere in the economy. Furthermore, given a choice among the recipients of alternative medical programs, the tendency will be for higher benefits (at equivalent costs, especially in curative programs for the same disease) to occur in treating wealthier groups. There are relatively low economic benefits to treating the unemployed, given this wage-equals-social-value approach. However, economists argue, cost-benefit analysis is only supposed to give one an idea of which investment is more efficient, not more equitable. It is typically claimed that the value of the technique is to explicitly quantify the benefit or loss in social efficiency from public decisions. This efficiency result in cost-benefit analysis is predicated on the existence of competitive markets for all inputs and all outputs.

The above questions concerning the use of economic analysis in making health status decisions cause problems even when the assumptions of economic analysis hold. However, when markets are not perfectly competitive, prices do not represent social value. Economists sometimes attempt to estimate the true social cost (called "shadow price") of a system's inputs and outputs and still use cost-benefit analysis to determine efficiency. However, equity issues remain a critical problem. For example, economists have viewed the American Medical Association in the United States as an organization that, in effect, restricts the supply of medical personnel, yielding higher incomes for those allowed into the medical profession and higher costs for curative services than would be found in a competitive system. Even if "true" competitive market prices could be estimated to evaluate a particular health program, the actual prices paid for doctors and services would result in doctors receiving more than their marginal product; in effect, this is a transfer of wealth from patients to doctors over and above what the latter's services are worth. Again, economic analysis generally ignores such equity considerations, arguing that they can be treated separately, if greater equity is considered socially desirable, through a governmental wealth-redistribution mechanism. By doing this, economists attempt to isolate their market criterion of efficiency as a relatively objective one that does not depend on the more subjective assessment by public sector decision makers of the society's preferences for equality. Unfortunately for this way of thinking, few if any economies operate according to the assumptions of the perfectly competitive system, and therefore, even within its own terms, cost-benefit analysis will not provide an accurate guide to social efficiency.

Given the problems above, many might state that the application of cost-benefit analysis to health evaluation is inequitable at best, and perhaps, in many ways, inhumane. However, some economists would likely respond that without looking at hard questions of the monetary costs and benefits of a health program, alternative social investments may be selected that would appear to be a better use of society's scarce resources. If decision makers wish to argue that considerations of humanity and equity demand a certain minimal worldwide level of health and nutrition regardless of the economic consequences of this investment, cost-effectiveness analysis may be sufficient for their purposes. However, most economists would assert that it is worthwhile for decision makers to consider economic benefits as well. In the remainder of this section, we focus on those health- and nutrition-related factors that economists usually examine when studying productivity. We will defer our discussion of the relationship of these factors to economic growth until Chapter 6. A discussion of the empirical methods that economists use to establish the causal impact of a factor or set of factors will be undertaken in Chapter 8.

Productivity change may be thought of as related to health in two ways: through direct effects (that is, healthier workers will have lower absenteeism, higher on-the-job capabilities, and greater life-span) and through indirect effects (that is, healthier persons will have

FIGURE 5.5

Model of the Nutrition-Productivity Relationship

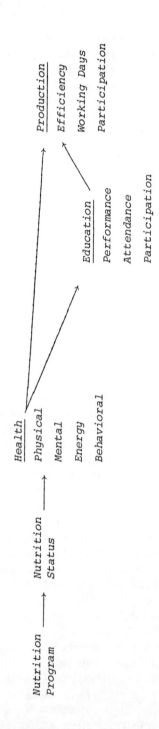

Source: Adapted from Cesario, Simon, and Kinne 1970. Reprinted by permission.

the capacity to learn more and thus to produce more). A model of the relationship of nutrition to productivity was provided by Cesario, Simon, and Kinne (1970). This model, showing direct and indirect effects, is adapted in schematic form in Figure 5.5.

Several studies have demonstrated the direct connection between health and nutrition status and productivity of workers. Many of the studies analyzed gave different diets to groups of workers to test their productivity in physical labor. Studies in which diets were altered for workers engaged in mental tasks were not available, although there are considerable numbers of studies linking nutrition in early childhood to brain development (see, for example, Sagan 1977; Cravioto and Robles 1965; Cravioto and DeLicardie 1968; Monckeberg 1968; Childers 1969; Guzman 1968; Coursin 1963; Stoch and Smythe 1968).

Malenbaum (1970) reported that agricultural output was related to health. In his study, he determined the effects of agricultural labor, commercial fertilizer, infant mortality, physician-population ratio, and illiteracy on agricultural output using linear regression analysis. He found that the two health-related variables explained 79 percent of the variance in agricultural output. However, Malenbaum improperly used health input and output measures, and the validity and generality of his results are suspect. In his study, infant mortality, a health output, and physician-population ratio, a health input, are both treated as independent variables affecting agricultural output. An equation first showing the relationship of health inputs to health outputs should have been estimated.

In studies of nutrition, Lele (1975) reported on a study discussed by Kraut and Muller (1946) conducted in Nazi Germany in which the raising of the caloric consumption of 20 workmen increased the dumping of materials from 1.5 tons per hour to 2.2 tons per hour. The original caloric consumption of these individuals had been 2,500 calories per day, and it was increased by 500 calories. Florencis and Evenson (unpublished) reported on an experiment that removed food from 32 male "volunteers." They were placed on a six-month semi-starvation diet. Those with a 15 percent weight loss had a 50 percent productivity decrease and a 30 percent decrease in ability to perform prolonged work. Those with a 50 percent weight loss experienced decreases of 90 percent and 80 percent, respectively. Florencis and Evenson also reported that the volunteers lacked self-discipline and tended to be nervous and lethargic. Winslow (1951) reported that an improvement in work productivity was experienced in building the Pan-American Highway when improved diets resulted in a tripling of paving. Correa (1968) reported that the working capacity of the labor force in India and El Salvador was only 50 percent of the normal level. Comparing developed with developing countries, he felt that it was reasonable to assume that nutrition would increase productivity.

In studies of the relationship of disease to productivity, Basta and Churchill (1974) reported a 20 percent increase in productivity when workers with anemia were given elemental iron at a cost of $0.31 per person per day. Because hookworm affects 600 million persons a year and is a major cause of anemia, they felt that preventive measures to eliminate hookworm could be more beneficial than treating the symptoms of anemia. Gilbert and Jones (1976) also analyzed the relationship between hookworm, poor diet, anemia, and work productivity. They felt that long-range, cost-benefit analysis indicated higher income from overall programs, including iron pills, building of latrines, wearing shoes, nutrition education, and antihookworm pills. Winslow (1951) reported that malaria resulted in an absenteeism of 25 percent in the Philippines. When attempts made to eliminate malaria reduced the absenteeism to between 2 and 4 percent, productivity increased and there was a need for 25 percent fewer workers. This situation could result in tremendous unemployment problems if the economy were not structured to absorb persons in alternative occupations. In a similar study of the eventual problematic impacts of disease reduction, Malenbaum (1973) reported that an increase in unemployment occurred when a UN program in Mexico reduced lead intoxication of pottery workers and improved their health, thus leading to expanded output.

Farooq (1964) analyzed several studies of schistosomiasis and reported a productivity decrease of 35 percent for infected workers. On the other hand, Foster (1967) reported no productivity decrease on an East African sugarcane estate for workers suffering schistosomiasis. However, according to most accounts, schistosomiasis is a particularly debilitating disease affecting 200 million persons throughout the world (Wen-Pin Chang 1971), and the major need is for preventive programs.

Analyses showing a direct connection between health and nutrition and productivity are concerned with the economic impact of working adults. In order to use cost-benefit analysis to justify investments in health, more complicated models are needed to link the indirect health and nutrition inputs to productivity. These indirect models are especially important for evaluating investments in nutrition and health for mothers and children.

A model for linking the nutrition of children to the productivity of adults was reported in Selowsky (1971, 1973) and Selowsky and Taylor (1971). The basic model may be summarized as a series of four equations, as follows: (1) earning = f (schooling, adult ability, socioeconomic status [SES]), (2) schooling = f (initial ability, SES), (3) adult ability = f (initial ability, SES, schooling), and (4) initial ability = f (nutrition, SES). These equations are represented in terms of a path model in Figure 5.6.

FIGURE 5.6

Path Model for Rate of Return of Infant Nutrition

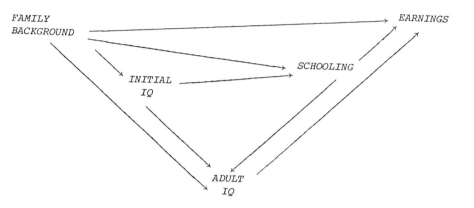

Unfortunately, an experimental group was not followed from infancy to adulthood in order to estimate the relationships in the equations. Two different groups were used in Chile to estimate the four equations: 40 children (for equation 4) and 90 construction workers, 30 employed and 60 unemployed (for equations 1, 2, 3). Using weight as a proxy for nutrition, Selowsky and Taylor reported an association between IQ and weight (other studies have shown a relationship between weight, physical size, and nutrition levels). From the analysis of construction workers, they found a positive relationship between initial IQ and adult IQ and between adult IQ and earnings. Interestingly, the employed construction workers had less schooling than the unemployed. By calculating the impacts of weight on initial IQ, initial IQ on adult IQ, and adult IQ on earnings, they were able to calculate an increase in earnings for an increase in weight. Assuming that the weight deficiencies could be compensated in the first two years of the child's life, they calculated a rate of return of 20 percent to the milk program. (Sorkin [1974] reported a similar rate of return for primary education in Chile.) The rate of return was calculated by an internal rate of return procedure where the discounted benefits of additional earnings from ages 15 to 45 were compared with the discounted costs of the milk for the child until age two.

The type of analysis suggested by Selowsky and Taylor is probably the best one could hope for from a cost-benefit approach. Yet, there are many faults with the analysis. Sorkin (1976) suggested that the rate of return was underestimated, since several benefits were excluded from the analysis, including: (1) increased earnings one normally expects from schooling (their data would have indicated a decrease), (2) savings in medical costs owing to a reduction of illness, and (3) general income increases to the poor because of a potential change in income distribution. However, one could argue that there are several reasons for an overestimation of benefits. First, there is considerable controversy over the validity of IQ testing. Jensen (1969) argued that IQ was mostly hereditary; Bowles and Gintis (1973) argued that IQ was a function of social class. If either of these arguments is substantially correct, IQ may not help to measure the relationship between nutrition and brain development. This relationship, as we have reported, has been substantiated by several studies of children in their early years. Additionally, brain development is more closely related to protein consumption than to caloric consumption. Thus, the relationship between body weight and IQ is highly questionable as a surrogate for the relationship between protein deficiency and intellectual capacity.

Furthermore, it is questionable whether the size of the differences observed in IQ has as much of an impact on earnings as unmeasured worker characteristics. There is considerable controversy regarding the effect of education on earnings. This controversy may be extended to IQ. Several economists (for example, Schultz 1961, 1963; Weisbrod 1962; Becker 1964) have reported direct relationships between education and additional earnings. However, others (for example, Gintis 1971) have argued that the relationship between education and earnings does not reflect on the intrinsic value of education or a person's ability to learn but, rather, on a person's ability to operate according to the rules of the school structure (such as promptness and responsiveness to authoritarian, hierarchical power structures). It is the process of schooling rather than the content that prepares individuals for their place in the work world. Alternatively, schooling structure and content may not teach anything of value but simply serve as a "screening" selection mechanism, as some economists have suggested (for example, Arrow 1973; Spence 1973). This screening mechanism may be associated with IQ, but higher IQ does not increase likelihood of selection. Thus, even though IQ is associated with earnings, it may not be possible to improve earnings by raising IQ.

Another problem with the analysis of Selowsky and Taylor (1971) is that they considered as costs only the price of the milk. Costs to administer the program and distribute the milk were ignored. Additionally, it would be necessary to ensure that the free milk were not used by families as a substitute for purchased food, thus resulting in no improvement in the child's health. A health education program in conjunction with the free milk program could be crucial to ensure its success. The costs of such a health education program would have to be included in the cost-benefit analysis.

The last and perhaps the most fundamental problem of any long-term, rate-of-return analysis for employment is the marginality of the analysis. A rate-of-return analysis is only accurate—if it is accurate at all—for the next person employed (the individual at the margin). Increasing the labor force by one person or increasing the health of one laborer would have little impact on the wages paid to laborers. However, massive changes, such as a free milk program to all children, may have no effect or even a detrimental effect on individual earnings, since the labor market would be flooded with more capable, healthier workers: rather than raising wages, employers might respond by raising the qualifications required for additional income or even by lowering wages. Similar problems hold for rate-of-return analysis of education. For example, a country may choose a large investment in secondary education based upon the higher wages earned by persons with secondary education in the current labor market. However, when secondary education is implemented on a large scale, it is found that employment formerly available to persons with secondary education now requires a college diploma. The country may then find that the investment in education has increased the education level of the unemployed, as happened in India (Blaug, Layard, and Woodhall 1969).

Given the data problems of a long-term rate-of-return study and the questionable validity of such a model, the analysis pursued by Selowsky and Taylor (1971) is the best one could hope to accomplish —and even this has very serious problems, as we have seen. One motivation for attempting this type of mathematical analysis of a process, such as relating infant nutrition to lifetime employment, is the alleged desire by planners for quantification. Cesario, Simon, and Kinne (1970), Berg (1973), and David and Omran (1974), among others, felt that planners would tend to choose those projects for which a detailed quantification of benefits and costs was available. Without this analysis, it was felt that infant nutrition would be ignored. Programs that satisfy basic societal priorities but lack quantification should not be rejected when such quantification leads analysts to resort to "statistical sleight of hand to apply theory to inadequate data" (Selowsky and Taylor 1971).

Perhaps the simplest cost-benefit approach to apply (given a willingness to accept monetary values as a valid measure of social costs and benefits) is that with any study of nutrition or health in which the benefits are a savings of other medical costs or an immediate increase in days worked. For example, Sorkin (1976) claimed that Selowsky and Taylor had underestimated benefits by ignoring the immediate benefits of reduced treatment costs for children if improved nutrition decreased disease incidence.

A similar approach was reported for a cost-benefit study of the "barefoot doctors" in China (Sorkin 1976). The barefoot doctors are agricultural persons with some medical training who have a primary responsibility to health education and preventive medicine (Smith 1974). These persons receive a wage of $120 per year, equivalent to a typical peasant wage (Seidel 1972). Benefits of the barefoot doctor system include: (1) reductions in workdays lost owing to illness and (2) reductions in travel time to obtain service when health assistance is not immediately available. The costs of the system include: (1) providing and receiving training and (2) providing and receiving the service. The time required of all participants—patients, barefoot doctors (in training and dispensing service), and trainers—is included in the analysis. The benefit to cost ratios ranged from 3:1 to 5:1 in the four provinces studied.

The quantitative techniques discussed in this chapter are replete with problems. The most important common characteristic is that the air of objectivity given to the analysis through detailed numerical manipulation has little substance. The manner in which a model is formulated and the type of data chosen for inclusion and exclusion reflect the subjectivity of the analyst. A fundamental subjectivity reflected in cost-benefit analysis, in particular, is that economically measurable benefits derived from the price system are of primary importance. This philosophy is a reflection of an orientation toward economic growth, the assumption being that high growth rates lead to a social opportunity to improve the standard of living for all citizens, as measured by the value of material goods production. Theoretically, the creation of more income and more employment opportunities should result in improved nutrition and health. In the next chapter, we discuss in detail some models linking health and nutrition to GNP growth and some of the impacts of growth on health.

6
HEALTH, EDUCATION, AND ECONOMIC GROWTH

MODELS OF ECONOMIC GROWTH

Gross national product (GNP) is the most commonly used measure of the value of all goods and services produced in the economy. A growth in GNP can occur either because more goods and services are produced or because the value of those produced has increased. According to Nader, Green, and Seligman (1976), corporate production increases GNP in two ways: through the value of the goods produced and the value of the resources needed to negate the effects of pollution. Therefore, as spending to combat pollution and to give medical care increases, the GNP increases. GNP accounts also include repairs for negligence and waste disposal. All these apparently negative activities are included in GNP accounts because each provides employment and payment to other resource inputs. Paradoxically, then, a health project that has a favorable cost-benefit ratio may reduce GNP if the major benefit measured is a savings in medical care costs. In theory, an adequate GNP measure should subtract the costs of many of these activities as inputs to the quality of life. The justification for a health project investment that reduces medical treatment costs is that the savings in health care resources would allow those resources to be utilized in other productive endeavors, and GNP would be only marginally effected. (This assumes that resources are allocated to their "best" use and that a reallocation would be to a "second best" use.)

Because it increases prices, inflation may be a major contributory factor in growth of GNP. Therefore, the attempt is made to calculate the "real" GNP by adjusting the "nominal" GNP (goods and services multiplied by current prices) by a price index. This price index is constructed for a representative bundle of goods purchased in society by both businesses and consumers. Calculating this price index as an

73

adjustment mechanism for GNP implicitly assumes that all factors that affect supply and demand for different goods will be ignored. Consumer tastes may change because of increased advertising or changes in income, education, and health. These taste changes lead to a shift in the market demand curve and consequent changes in market prices. Price changes due to these changes are not inflationary and should not be used to adjust the GNP. However, since it is hard to attribute price changes to inflation changes (as opposed to market changes), it is assumed that all market changes balance. Thus, one is left only with inflationary price changes for the goods analyzed.

One other major fault with GNP accounting is that only quantities of goods and services are included. There is no accounting for changes in the quality of goods. For example, if wooden desks are included at all as a separate category, they are not further subdivided by quality. In time, the quality of a product may decline, while its price remains constant. However, the quality of the good has declined and this change would not be reflected in GNP. Additionally, and perhaps most important, the general quality of life is not considered by GNP. Job satisfaction or the psychological impacts of improved health are totally ignored.

The basic model used by economists explains GNP in the manner of a simple production function where the output, GNP, is a function of two basic inputs: labor and physical capital. Clearly, there are very different types of labor and capital. However, these differences tend to be ignored in models explaining economic growth, and an attempt is made to construct an index for each factor of production. Increases in GNP are then attributed to increases in capital or labor, which are due to growth in the amount of capital (through investment) and the amount of labor (through population growth). However, studies of economic growth in the United States by many economists attempting to relate economic growth (changes in GNP) to changes in labor and capital have resulted in a residual factor of growth not explained by growth rates of labor and/or capital.

The existence of this residual factor led economists to discuss the role of technological change in two forms: embodied and disembodied. Embodied technological change is an improved quality in the factor of production: improved technology in new equipment (for example, replacement of vacuum tubes by printed circuits) and improved health and education in labor. For example, Schultz (1960) and Denison (1962) attributed approximately 20 percent of economic growth over several decades to increased education. Disembodied technological change involves factors basically associated with increased creativity in the management of organizations and resources. These ideas for improving management may also be a reflection of increased education.

Health affects economic growth in several ways: improved health of employed persons leads to increased labor participation; improved health leads to increased education, which in turn increases economic growth; and improved health may lead to population growth and increased labor force participation. As an example of the latter, Mushkin (1962) estimated that the decline in mortality rates in the United States since 1900 had increased GNP by $60 billion in 1960, owing to 13 million additional workers. She calculated that declining mortality rates since 1920, which had led to an increase of 6 million workers, had increased GNP in 1960 by $28 billion.

The three effects of nutrition programs on productivity (and economic growth) were explicitly accounted for by Cesario, Simon, and Kinne (1970). The focal point of their discussion was the effect of nutrition programs. One could construct similar models for health programs. In Figure 6.1 we have modified their model to include health programs and the interaction between health and nutrition. Health and nutrition programs may include a wide variety of different projects, such as health and nutrition education, preventive measures, curative health facilities, agricultural and related programs to increase food supplies, and income redistribution or price subsidization to increase spending on nutrition and health care.

The model suggests several ways in which the cost-effectiveness of health and nutrition programs may be analyzed. Measures of effectiveness include: nutrition status, morbidity, mortality, population growth, and the various factors related to personal improvement, education, and education effects. The simplest and most commonly used measures for a cost-effectiveness analysis are nutrition status, mortality, morbidity, and population growth. Benefits can then be measured in terms of changes in GNP as expressed through improvements (efficiency) and increases (working days and participation) in the labor force.

The different ways that health and nutrition programs can lead to changes in GNP may be easily observed in the schematic of the model. Programs that lead to improvements in nutrition and decreases in mortality and morbidity of adults can lead to increased participation by those not currently working and increased working days for those employed. Additionally, improvements in nutrition and health of employed adults can increase their working efficiency on the job through improvements in personal attributes. The impacts of health and nutrition programs on the young in terms of future GNP occur through changes in education. Reductions in morbidity and mortality can increase attendance and performance in educational institutions. However, as we have already pointed out, the connection between education and improved GNP is not clear. The final effects of improved health and nutrition occur through increased population

FIGURE 6.1

Disaggregated Policy Model Relation Health to GNP

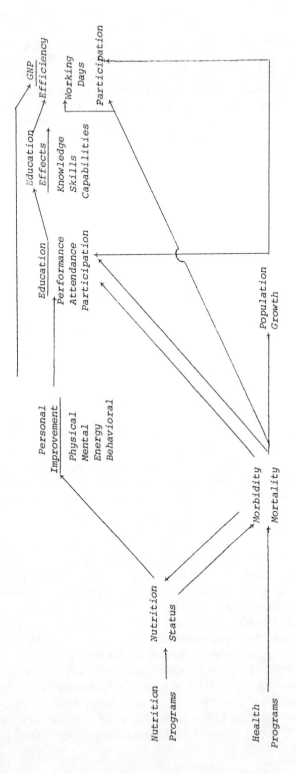

growth, which directly affects GNP through labor force participation rates and, indirectly, through increased education participation rates. However, increased population growth can have deleterious effects on GNP (see "Negative Aspect of the Health-GNP Interrelationship," below).

The model presented in Figure 6.1 is incomplete. Zukin (1975) included an important feedback loop from GNP increases to improved nutrition and reduced morbidity and mortality. This important aspect of economic growth can occur through increased personal income or spending on nutrition and health programs by government agencies. Jordan (1977) called this the traditional view of a trickle-down effect of improved living standards (including health) as economic growth continued. The expectation that rising GNP will raise health standards by encouraging government spending is questioned by Kleiman (1974). He claims that government spending is inefficient and, more important, that the reduced health spending caused by taxation of middle- and higher-income groups will not be balanced by new government spending for lower-income groups.

The proposition that health benefits will be derived from economic growth, as represented by the missing feedback loop in Figure 6.1, is at the heart of the divergence of views between those who analyze the structure in which decisions take place and those who analyze disaggregated policy decisions. The model in Figure 6.1 represents the latter view.

The impression given by the model is that if new health or nutrition programs are successful, GNP will increase. Every link in the model involves the influence of the societal structure and the socio-economic status of the participants. As we have pointed out earlier, the effect of any health or nutrition program on nutrition status, morbidity, and mortality is likely to be contingent on education or the availability of other resources. More fundamentally, however, one needs to examine the allocation of resources to different groups and regions in the country. The general tendency, which is being reversed in very few countries, is toward expensive curative facilities. Resource availability for massive health and nutrition programs is generally limited.

The impression that reductions in morbidity and mortality of adults and increases in population can lead to increased labor force participation is predicated on certain assumptions regarding industrial structures. Large, concentrated firms biased toward capital-intensive investment will not provide job openings to accommodate all new workers. The effect of an increased labor force may be an increase in the number of unemployed, a depression of wages given the larger number of people competing for jobs, and little effect on GNP.

The impression that improved health and nutrition and increased population growth will increase participation, attendance, and performance in educational institutions is based upon the belief that educational opportunities are available but not acted upon by individuals because of their ill health. There are many social forces that keep the healthy child out of school. These forces include the need for additional family income, the lack of educational opportunity for many beyond primary school, and the irrelevance of centrally controlled urban-based curricula for rural areas.

Improved health makes possible an increase in education, but only if there is at the same time a commitment of resources to expanding educational opportunities. Though improved educational opportunities may augment the knowledge, skills, and behavior of individuals, this improvement will not be translated into jobs if the expansion of the educated labor force causes a rise in the qualification levels for existing jobs rather than an increase in new jobs created. Additionally, there is the possibility that employers view schooling as a device to differentiate among students according to the school attended, using noneducational factors related to success in schooling rather than learning.

EVIDENCE OF A POSITIVE
RELATIONSHIP BETWEEN HEALTH AND GNP

Despite the potential problems of the disaggregated model ignoring the social context in which educational investments may take place, there are many empirical studies indicating that GNP increases can occur through the eradication of disease. The impact of disease eradication can most easily be seen in the opening of new land.

Kamarck (1976) reported on several diseases in Africa. Trypanosomiasis (sleeping sickness), which killed horses and cattle, led to increased reliance on humans for moving materials and for accomplishing the necessary physical labor involved in planting and harvesting. Thus, the essential first step in labor saving in agriculture has been ruled out. Additionally, trypanosomiasis has rendered one-third of Africa unsuitable for cattle raising and has aggravated protein deficiency problems. The threat of parasitic infection and fear of onchocerciasis (river blindness) has kept humans out of many fertile land areas. Nash (1974) discussed the benefits of a malaria eradication project in Nepal that opened fertile valleys to agricultural development. Before these areas were made available, mountain slopes were used. The latter were harder to cultivate and provided lower yields for a given labor input.

Correa and Cummins (1970) investigated the contribution of increased caloric intake and education to GNP growth for selected countries from 1950 to 1962. The results are summarized in Table 6.1.

TABLE 6.1

Contribution of Caloric Consumption and Education
to Economic Growth

Country	Economic Growth Rate (1950–62)	Percentage Contribution of Caloric Consumption	Percentage Contribution of Education
Latin America			
Average	5.13	4.6	5.4
Argentina	3.19	0.0	16.5
Brazil	5.43	4.2	3.3
Chile	4.20	1.2	4.8
Colombia	4.79	6.4	4.1
Ecuador	4.72	0.0	4.9
Honduras	4.52	9.1	6.5
Mexico	5.97	10.1	0.8
Peru	5.63	7.6	—
Venezuela	7.74	2.4	2.4
Europe and the United States			
Average	4.18	0.8	7.9
Belgium	3.20	0.6	13.4
Denmark	3.51	0.0	4.0
France	4.92	1.0	5.9
Germany	7.26	2.2	1.5
Italy	5.96	2.7	6.7
Netherlands	4.73	0.0	5.1
Norway	3.45	0.0	0.0
United Kingdom	2.29	0.4	12.7
United States	3.32	0.0	14.8

Source: Correa and Cummins (1970). Reprinted by permission.

A comparison of Latin America with Europe and the United States shows that the estimated contribution of growth to increased caloric consumption is higher in the Latin American countries (an average 4.6 percent of GNP growth in Latin America and 0.8 percent of GNP growth in the developed countries) and that the estimated growth contributed by education is lower (5.4 percent of GNP growth in Latin

America compared with 7.9 percent in developed countries). The first finding may support the argument that poor nutritional levels have restricted growth in developing countries. Additionally, these results indicate that the indirect effects of improving health for children, and consequently of increasing education, are important, since the contribution of education to growth (although lower than for developed countries) has a higher effect on growth in Latin America than does increased caloric consumption.

Another important aspect of the relationship of health to GNP is population growth. Mushkin (1962) discussed the large increases in GNP in the United States resulting from population growth. The model in Figure 6.1 also shows positive benefits of population growth on GNP. However, as Sorkin (1976) pointed out, it is GNP growth per capita that is important to present well-being and future growth potential. Rising GNP per capita allows new capital investment to take place and results in further economic growth. Therefore, while rising population may increase total GNP, the same increase in population may hinder future economic growth by restricting capital availability. Sorkin (1976) analyzed several countries to determine how much investment would be required to maintain a constant GNP per capita. He compared this needed demographic investment with actual capital formation to determine the amount available for expansionary capital investment. His analysis is reported in Table 6.2. Higher population growth rates of developing countries (2.5 times that in the developed countries) and lower rates of capital formation (70 percent of that in developed countries) result in much higher proportions of capital formation required to maintain current GNP per capita levels (42.5 percent of capital formation in developing countries and 12.5 percent of capital formation in developed countries).

The implication of Sorkin's analysis is that countries are better off with reduced, rather than increased, population growth. While it is apparent that diminished population growth will increase GNP per capita, the distributional effects are unclear. Much of the gain in increased GNP per capita could be concentrated in a relatively small group of society. However, the possibility of a distributed gain may be higher with a restricted population growth than without it. Weisbrod (1971) suggested that cost-benefit analysis be utilized to reflect the effect of population growth on GNP. While he agreed that the benefits of reduced morbidity and mortality included increased production, he argued that the production benefits should be reduced by increases in individual consumption. He viewed increased consumption as a drain on social resources that would reduce investment opportunities. The argument that population growth restricts new economic growth is based upon a capital investment model of economic development. It is not at all clear that capital investment is the most important ele-

TABLE 6.2

Percentage of Capital Formation Required to Maintain Current GNP per Capita

Country	Rate of Population Growth, 1965–70	Required Demographic Investment, Percentage of GNP	Rate of Capital Formation, 1966–68	Demographic Investment as a Percentage of Capital Format
Developing countries				
Overall	2.4	7.2	17.4	42.5
India	2.6	7.8	16.5	47.3
Indonesia	2.9	8.7	8.8	98.9
Brazil	2.8	8.4	17.2	48.8
Bangladesh	3.0	9.0	12.3	73.2
Pakistan	3.2	9.6	14.3	67.1
Nigeria	2.5	7.5	12.3	61.0
Mexico	3.4	10.2	15.6	65.4
Developed countries				
Overall (nonsocialist)	1.0	3.0	24.0	12.5
France	0.9	2.7	25.4	10.6
West Germany	0.6	1.8	24.3	7.4
Japan	1.1	3.3	32.9	10.0
United Kingdom	0.5	1.5	19.0	7.9
United States	1.1	3.3	16.7	19.8

Source: Sorkin (1976). Reprinted by permission.

ment of growth, since models of growth include both changes in capital and embodied technological progress in the labor force. It is quite possible that growth based upon labor-intensive investments may be more beneficial to developing countries.

NEGATIVE ASPECT OF THE
HEALTH-GNP INTERRELATIONSHIP

A major negative impact of health improvement on GNP may be the deterioration of the quality of life as a consequence of population growth. Many authors (for example, Ruchlin and Rogers 1973; Sorkin 1976; Jordan 1977) have argued that a primary impact of health improvement is a reduction in infant and adult mortality. Fewer adult deaths may have the short-term effect of increased unemployment. Fewer infant deaths will likely result in increased population growth, even if it is assumed that the high birthrates in developing countries are based to a large extent on expected infant deaths. There is likely to be a lagged response to a realization that diminished infant mortality rates are a permanent change and that fewer births are needed. The high population growth is due to this delayed response in reducing births. Ruchlin and Rogers (1973) felt that economic growth would be inhibited, since the increased population growth would increase the dependency ratio (the ratio of nonworking persons to working persons) and reduce the availability of savings. In fact, this increased dependency ratio resulting from health improvements and lower mortality rates would have potentially negative effects if given budgets for health and education were divided by increasing numbers of people. Furthermore, they felt that the decreased health spending per capita would eventually reduce the productivity of labor. Therefore, although population increase would increase GNP, the negative secondary effects could lead to a zero or negative change in GNP per capita. Barlow (1967), in a study of Ceylon, supported this analysis when he stated that the halving of mortality rates in Ceylon led to a doubled population growth that could eventually lead to diminished GNP per capita.

There are also negative impacts of economic growth on health problems. Sorkin (1976) thought that the increased urbanization resulting from economic growth would magnify health problems, especially in terms of sanitation and water availability. Reutlinger and Selowsky (1976) asserted that economic growth could diminish infant nutrition, since working mothers would stop breast-feeding babies and a substantial portion of their incomes would have to be allocated to infant nutrition to compensate for lost nutrients. The decline in breast-feeding may result in major economic problems in developing countries. Jelliffe and Jelliffe (1977) maintained that the main cause of the decline was urbanization, modernization, and advertising pressure from multinational corporations to purchase substitutes. They discussed the much-publicized "Nestle Kills Babies" case, in which Nestle's won slander charges and nominal payment but the judge warned that Nestle's "should carry out a fundamental reconsideration of its sales techniques in less developed countries . . . if it does not want its products to become lethally dangerous." Berg (1973) and Jelliffe and Jelliffe (1975) stated that food substitution (for breast-feeding) would place a substantial strain on family resources and lead to the purchase of foods that would contribute to death, disease, and poor physical health for nonnursing infants. Additionally, food substitution might increase population growth, since lactation inhibits pregnancy (Buchanan 1975).

Economic growth can be seen to have negative health effects even in more advanced countries. Eyer and Sterling (1977) argued that the stress created in capitalist societies through competition for jobs, unemployment, and alienation from work increased deaths and diseases in the United States. They stated that the effects of stress were more prevalent among the young and were more noticeable among the poor.

Sorkin (1976) cited several studies that indicated a negative effect of economic development on health. Scott (1957) investigated trypanosomiasis in West Africa and found that disease incidence was increased in adult males as a result of migration for work. Thus, highways linking countries also provide a channel for transmission of disease. El-Nazar (1958) reported that migrant workers from West Africa had brought schistosomiasis into the Sudan.

Development projects have similarly increased disease. Apted, et al. (1963) reported that a dam project in Rhodesia had resulted in the migration of an entire tribe from their fertile lands to dryer lands where they were unable to grow traditional crops. Additionally, they lost the protein source that they had in the fish from the lake in the dam region. Serious malnutrition resulted from this forced move. The problem was amplified by an outbreak of trypanosomiasis caused by the location of a government store that distributed grain.

The spread of schistosomiasis has also been linked to development projects and migratory labor (Hughes and Hunter 1970; Waddy 1966; Lanoix 1958). Dam and irrigation projects provide a natural environment for snails that carry the disease. Migratory workers who come to work in these irrigated areas may be infected and cause the disease to spread. However, it should be realized that though this irrigation has increased the number of snails that lead to infection, the problem is exacerbated by unsanitary habits on the part of migrant workers and by a lack of sanitary facilities.

In conclusion, population growth and certain health changes may hinder economic development and even promote a reduction in the health status of a population. Nonetheless, health programs may foster economic growth in some areas, as has been indicated by a variety of studies. Many health problems can be traced to a lack of knowledge regarding appropriate sanitation methods, food preparation methods, and nutrition.

In the following chapter we examine specific economic considerations in choosing among alternative technologies that may be employed to organize and deliver health and nutrition education services.

7
COMMUNICATION STRATEGIES
FOR HEALTH IMPROVEMENT

THE ROLE OF COMMUNICATIONS IN HEALTH

To reduce health problems in developing countries, one may adopt long- or short-term solutions. Long-term solutions attack the basic cause of health problems: poverty. There is considerable agreement throughout the literature on health that low income is correlated with low education and low health status. Low-income levels reduce the ability of parents to raise the health and education levels of their children, who, in turn, mature to find themselves in low-income positions. Advocates of private ownership of capital conclude that standards of living for the entire population improve when the economic climate is amenable to private investment and business growth. Opponents of this viewpoint range widely. There are those who argue that large corporations, though essential for economic growth, cannot solve all social problems and that government expenditures must be used for these problems. Others accept private ownership only on a small scale (they oppose concentrated, large-scale domestic and multinational corporations), combined with a system of government expenditures. Still others surmise that large corporations are an inevitable outgrowth of a system that supports private ownership and that for meaningful global development to begin, the existing capitalist structures must be changed. While government expenditures for health are seen, in the first two viewpoints, to have some effect on health status of the population, in the latter viewpoint such reforms will, in essence, maintain the status quo and cannot be expected to have far-reaching effects. These reforms are thought to delay the considerable social reorganization needed to yield significant changes in health and other aspects of social welfare. Such reorganization would include reducing corporate power, which, as we discussed earlier, contributes to major health problems that result from the pursuit of nonnutritious cash crop agriculture and the tendency to focus on the construction of a centralized, hierarchical, capital-intensive, curative health system.

In effect, shorter-term solutions to health problems accept the structural status quo and formulate programs directed toward some of the more harmful symptoms. Following the model of Figure 6.1, these health intervention strategies may have long-term benefits in economic growth. Simple and relatively inexpensive sanitation and health practices can inhibit the spread of disease. Assuming that food is available, an understanding of nutritional needs can help to reduce malnutrition and diseases related to it. Programs aimed at changing health, sanitation, or nutritive practices almost always involve an education component in addition to any related program to ensure the availability of resources.

Since most of these health education programs will be directed toward adults who are no longer part of the formal school system and who may be illiterate, communications technology is being used with increasing frequency to disperse health education information. Communications technology systems have been used for a wide variety of educational purposes throughout the world (Wells 1976; Schramm 1977). The main benefits are access to large portions of the population, relatively low cost, and uniformity and quality of program content. There are also potential negative effects, such as centralization of program content and associated control, the capital-intensive nature of the investment, and the reliance on foreign nations for physical and human resources for implementation and programming. Centralized message control may have disastrous effects when an error is made: in Nicaragua (Manoff 1976; Cooke and Romweber 1977), a radio script, when translated into Spanish, had the wrong proportion of ingredients for a curative mixture for diarrhea and could have resulted in death from excess salt intake. Additionally, information on health practices dispersed through mass media may appear to lend credence to corporate advertising that promotes poor health practices. Jelliffe and Jelliffe (1977) blamed the dominance of mass media and corporate advertising for contributing to a major decline in breast-feeding and a consequent change to marketed products that require large portions of low-income budgets to provide sufficient nutrition as a substitute. McKigney (1968) also analyzed this trend toward early weaning and concluded that it was partly a result of the economic necessity for women to work reinforced by exposure to "modern" ideas and tastes through inappropriate advertising. This switch to corporate-produced food is frequently accompanied by severe malnutrition and diarrhea in children, since the powdered milk products are often over-diluted. While communications technology-health education programs may accomplish the specific learning objectives established for them, the credibility carried over to commercial mass media use can have strongly negative effects.

THE EVALUATION OF COMMUNI-
CATIONS TECHNOLOGY SYSTEMS

Several factors must be considered in applying the restricted quantitative techniques of cost, cost-effectiveness, and cost-benefit analysis to the choice of a communications technology system that functions as part of a health education strategy. (Klees and Wells [1977] discussed the latter two techniques for instructional technology systems applied in any educational setting.) Although the basic methodological approach to cost analysis is unaffected, the manner in which costs are treated may differ under certain circumstances. For example, it is unlikely that health education programs will completely utilize the capacity of a communications system. A radio channel that covers a region or all regions of a country will have a maximum capacity of 24 hours, seven days a week. However, given audience working and sleeping hours, the practical hourly capacity for health education programs may be reduced to only a few hours each day. Mass media communications technology systems such as radio and television usually have relatively high initial investment in equipment and facilities for production and transmission. If the system is to be used only for health education projects, all equipment and facility expenses should be allocated to the health education programs. However, when a communications system is constructed for multiple purposes or when time on an existing station is made available for health education programs, there are no fixed rules on cost allocation. One may allocate costs on the basis of time devoted to different programs or by considering health education a marginal addition to the communications system. In the latter approach one considers the equipment and facilities as "sunk" costs; that is, the decision to implement the health education program has no effect on the investment costs. One would consider only the specific operating and maintenance costs associated with the health education system.

Costs for education systems are often reported on the basis of average cost per student. In order to determine total costs, one needs to know the number of participants and be able to calculate costs for participant time and for radio batteries and receivers. However, levels of participation in mass media health education programs are hard to determine when such participation is informal.

The cost information that is most readily available to decision makers is total costs for facilities and equipment for production and transmission, hourly operation costs for equipment, and hourly production costs. Decision makers tend to ignore other costs. However, from the social cost viewpoint, which considers all resources, one would also calculate costs based on assumptions for average wages (as a measure of opportunity cost), radio batteries, and radio receiver cost. (However, on the assumption that receivers will not be purchased for the health program, this latter cost is often treated as a sunk cost and only additional maintenance is included.) One may then derive a total cost function for an instructional technology project, such as the one below:

$$TC = F + V_{ph}N_{ph} + V_{th}N_{th} + V_pN_p \qquad (7.1)$$

where TC = total cost;

F = fixed cost (that is, those costs, such as administration, that are invariant with respect to the other parameters in the equation);

V_{ph} = variable cost per production hour (that is, recurrent and annualized capital costs for all facilities, equipment, and personnel related to program production);

V_{th} = variable cost per transmission hour (that is, recurrent and annualized capital costs for all facilities, equipment, and personnel related to transmitting the program from the production source to the participants);

V_p = variable cost per participant (that is, time of participants, radio receivers, and, in some cases, all costs related to producing and distributing printed materials);

N_{ph} = the number of original programming hours;

N_{th} = the total number of transmission hours including repetitions; and

N_p = the total number of participants (however calculated).

Any government ministry deciding on whether the health education investment should be made would probably modify equation 7.1 to reflect only expenditures from its budget. From a social viewpoint, this modification would be incorrect, since all resources involved in the program would not be considered. A communications technology-health education program magnifies the possibility that some costs will be ignored, since responsibility and participation are often divided among ministries—such as health, education, and communications—each with different goals. Depending upon which ministry receives ultimate responsibility for the project, the costs to the other ministries will often be ignored.

The distinction between the perspectives of different ministries may become more pronounced when health education investments are being made. While one would infer from cost-benefit analysis that the appropriate social decision makers would compare costs and benefits for a variety of projects regardless of ministries, in practice each ministry is faced with allocation decisions for its own budget. Therefore, each ministry will compare an investment in a health education communications technology project with other specific projects within its sphere of influence. The health ministry will be concerned with other health programs, the education ministry with other education programs, and the communications ministry with other uses of communications facilities (in many cases, for propaganda purposes).

This potential separation among ministries also leads to a disaggregated planning policy, and most analyses (if they evaluate the project at all) only view educational effectiveness of the program, not health status changes. The reason for this apparently myopic view is that education evaluators often assume, implicitly or explicitly, that given the most cost-effective alternative for increase in knowledge, one can expect the most favorable cost-benefit outcome. It is assumed that the education alternative can only affect knowledge gained, attitudes, or, in some cases, behavior. The relationship between these educational outcomes and changes in health status is thought to be independent of the particular education alternative chosen. Furthermore, the relationship between health status change and measurable benefits, such as increased productivity, is seen as independent of the health education alternative. This reasoning has some validity. If improvements in health increase economic productivity, then the manner in which the health improvement is obtained should have little bearing on the relationship between health and growth.

Important factors that differentiate among health education strategies according to ultimate cost and benefit impacts are those items outside the framework of the original objectives. In the case of communications technology, those items include the creation of additional credibility for commercial advertising with potentially negative health effects, the foreign exchange problems resulting from the fact that most communications technology systems require imported equipment, and a continued reliance on centralized authority and information control that may restrict future local initiative for improvement. The last problem may be ameliorated somewhat by health campaigns, such as Tanzania's "Man Is Health" and "Food Is Life" programs, in which the centrally controlled radio system was used to initiate community and individual projects aimed at reducing health problems and increasing food supplies.

There is an additional problem in assessing the educational cost-effectiveness of a system. Oettinger and Zapol (1972) proposed that education systems could be arrayed on a spectrum from a relatively adaptable one-to-one, personal-contact system to standardized mass media that would be more formalized and less flexible. Accordingly, Green (1977a) concluded that the advantage of mass media was its economy of scale, that is, the ability to produce a unit of instruction and distribute it to a very large number of people. These economies of scale would considerably lower average costs for large numbers of participants and might have average effectiveness levels similar to more personalized approaches. In fact, studies of a wide range of instructional strategies indicate relatively few differences in effectiveness (see, for example, Jamison, Suppes, and Wells 1974).

SUMMARY OF COMMUNICATIONS
TECHNOLOGY PROJECTS

While economists have proposed increasing use of cost-effectiveness and cost-benefit analyses, education projects, particularly those involving communications technology, have tended to evaluate only educational outcomes. (An analysis of costs for several non-health-related communications technology projects in education was presented by Jamison, Klees, and Wells 1978.) Additionally, those health education projects that analyzed costs have used a wide variety of methods, and the results were not comparable. Leslie (1978b) summarized several health and nutrition education programs throughout the world. The results are shown in Table 7.1. These projects include nutrition education programs in the Philippines, Nicaragua, Trinidad and Tobago, Tanzania, Korea, India, Lesotho, and Micronesia, and health education projects in Kenya, Tanzania, Senegal, Haiti, Guatemala, and India. Of these 15 projects, 10 used radio (either alone or in combination with printed materials) and the remaining used film, television, or radio cassettes. The potential for lower average costs of radio programs is evident in the fact that the radio projects had far higher participation levels. All but one of the programs were directed toward adults, and five were directed toward mothers and pregnant women to encourage breast-feeding or health and nutrition practices for young children. None of the projects measured specific health effects, such as increases in nutrition status or decreases in mortality and morbidity, though several projects did measure behavioral changes. (Leslie considered these to be educational objectives.) It is presumed that these behavioral changes would lead to health status changes; otherwise, the objectives of the program —rather than the particular delivery system—should be faulted. These behavioral changes included: 7,500 mothers improving the nutritive value of weaning food in the Philippines (Cooke and Romweber 1977; Zeitlan and Formacion 1977); 17,500 mothers using a simple mixture to treat diarrhea in children in Nicaragua (Cooke and Romweber 1977); the construction of vegetable garden and poultry units in Tanzania

TABLE 7.1

Communications Technology Projects for Health and Nutrition Education

Name of Project	Description					Evaluation				References
	Country	Media	Duration	Target Audience	Major Message	Outreach	Educational Objectives	Health Objectives	Cost	
Manoff International Advertising Technique Nutrition Education Campaign	Philippines	Radio	A one-year campaign, October 1975 to October 1976	Mothers of children under 12 months	Enrich weaning food with oil, fish, and vegetables	50 to 75 percent (approximately 30,000 mothers) heard and remembered the message	10 to 25 percent mothers began enrichment of weaning food	No significant effects on the weight gain of children	$1.50 to $2.50 per mother reached	Zeitlan and Formacion 1977; Cooke and Romweber 1977
Manoff International Advertising Technique Nutrition Education Campaign	Nicaragua	Radio	A ten-month Campaign, 1976 to May 1977	Mothers of children five years old and under	Recipe given for Super Limonada for home rehydration of children with diarrhea	Approximately 65 percent (70,000 mothers) heard and remembered the message	Approximately 25 percent mothers gave Super Limonada for diarrhea	—	$0.65 to $1.75 per mother reached	Cooke and Romweber 1977
Trinidad and Tobago Breast-feeding Campaign	Trinidad and Tobago	Radio, television, newspaper	A six-week campaign in June and July 1974	Mothers and pregnant women	Breast-feeding is preferable to bottle feeding	75 to 99 percent of women recognized the messages from one or more media	Mothers with more awareness of the campaign introduced bottle feeding later	—	—	Gueri 1975
Food Is Life Campaign	Tanzania	Radio and booklet	A three-month campaign, June to September 1975	Rural adults	Produce and consume a variety of foods for better health	1.5 million to 3 million participants in radio-listening groups	Some new vegetable gardens and poultry units were begun	—	—	Mahai 1975; Matiko 1976
CARE Mass Media Nutrition Education Campaign	Korea	Radio and comic book	A one-year campaign, January to December 1970	All Korean adults	For good health, eat foods from each of the five food groups	70 to 80 percent heard or read the messages	20 percent could name nutrients supplied by the five food groups	—	—	Higgins and Montague 1972

(continued)

91

TABLE 7.1 (continued)

Name of Project	Description					Evaluation			References
	Country	Media	Duration	Target Audience	Major Message	Outreach	Educational Objectives	Health Objectives	Cost	
CARE Mass Media Nutrition Education Campaign	India	Film, poster, billboard, and radio	A ten-week campaign, April to June 1972	Mothers and pregnant women	The diet of a six-month-old child should include solid foods	250,000 people lived in the catchment area of the eight experimental sites	Awareness of recommended weaning behavior increased from 50 to 93 percent	–	–	Parlato 1974; Krishnamurthy 1976
Giving Birth and Caring for Your Children	Kenya	Radio	Weekly broadcasts, began in February 1975	Rural adults	A variety of modern child care practices are promoted in a dialogue comedy format	3 million listeners	–	–	$350.00 per show; $0.000 per listener	Hostetler 1976; Harris 1976
Man Is Health Campaign	Tanzania	Radio and booklet	Campaign during 1973	Rural adults	Recognition and prevention of malaria, hookworm, dysentery, bilharzia, and tuberculosis	1 million to 2 million participants in radio-listening groups	20 percent of groups built latrines (750,000 latrines)	–	$0.50 per villager reached	Matiko 1976; Hall and Dodds 1977
Social Education of Women	Senegal	Television	Broadcasts, began in March 1965	Illiterate working-class women in television clubs in Dakar	Information about the cause and treatment of malaria, dysentery, and tuberculosis and promotion of less use of oil for cooking	500 women regularly attended television club meetings twice a week	Recognition of mosquito as cause of malaria increased from 41 to 76 percent and use of more than seven liters of oil per week decreased from 61 to 15 percent	–	–	Fougeyrollas 1967
Class d'Hygiene	Haiti	Radio	A 12-week campaign repeated yearly, since 1970	Fifth- and sixth-grade schoolchildren and their teachers	Information on physiology, vaccination, and population growth	In 1974 there were approximately 3,500 participants from 194 different localities	–	–	–	Hollant 1977

92

Project	Country	Medium	Timing	Target audience	Message	Exposure	Results		Cost	Source
The Pila Communication Project	Guatemala	Audio cassette	Three-week campaign during 1975	Women on a coffee and rubber plantation	Promotion of vaccinations and consumption of Incaparina	Most women on the plantation heard the tapes	Experimental plantation had 92 percent rate for second vaccinations against polio and diphtheria compared with a 60 percent rate in a control plantation	—	$0.02 per household reached	Colle 1977; Clearinghouse on Development Communication 1977
Satellite Instructional Television Experiment (SITE)	India	Television	August 1975 to August 1976	Rural adults	Preventive medicine through improved nutrition and Ayurvedic herbal home remedies	400 villages in six states	Pre- to posttest gains of 20 to 40 percent on all health questions	—	—	Dighe and Roy 1977
Maharashtra State Mass Media Nutrition Education Campaign	India	Newspaper and film	A one-year campaign in the early 1970s	People with an income of at least Rs250 per month living in towns with at least 25,000 population	Good-quality protein should be part of the diet, especially for children	Approximately 53 percent (2.7 million adults) were aware of the campaign	20 to 30 percent reported changing their diet due to the campaign	—	$0.04 per contract	PAG Secretariat 1976
Lesotho Distance Teaching Centre Nutrition Campaign	Lesotho	Radio and comic book	A two-week campaign in November 1975	Rural women	Beans, green vegetables, and potatoes make a balanced diet for good health	10 to 30 percent of women in lowlands area (20,000 women) heard and remembered the radio spots	50 to 70 percent knew why each of the foods is good for health	—	—	Lesotho Distance Teaching Centre 1976
Yap District Nutrition Education Program	Micronesia	Filmstrip and radio spot	Project began in 1975	Mothers and pregnant women	Breast-feeding is more economical and better for infants than bottle feeding	500 to 1,000 women	Breast-feeding in clinic waiting rooms increased from 25 to 50 percent in two years	—	$0.02 to $0.05 per target woman	Rody 1978

Source: Leslie 1978b. Reprinted by permission.

93

(Mahai, et al. 1975; Matiko 1976); and the construction of 750,000 latrines in Tanzania (Matiko 1976; Hall and Dodds 1977). (See Chapter 9 below.)

In addition to the programs reported by Leslie (1978b), there has been considerable success reported in the use of mass media to promote birth control. Cuca and Pierce (1978) surveyed 96 experiments in family planning. They found that mass media combined with fieldwork (home visits or group meetings) significantly increased the acceptance rate of birth control practices. Sorkin (1976) reported similar results in that low-income families with high media exposure had 60 percent fewer births than low-income families with low media exposure. (Of course, a causal relationship is not ensured. See Chapter 8.)

The studies reported in Table 7.1 and those mentioned above indicate that communications technology can increase health knowledge and improve health practices. However, lack of consistency in cost and evaluation methodologies and the inability to prevent "control" groups from listening to experimental broadcasts reduces comparability among different projects and the ability to directly assign impacts to the technology program. These are two problems of research methodology. More fundamental problems are discussed in Chapter 8.

8
RESEARCH METHODOLOGY

Throughout this book we have cited numerous studies that rely on government statistics for health status and spending and other data manipulated in statistical models to reveal the effects of alternative educational systems on health knowledge and/or status, of health status on general education, of health status on productivity, and of education on productivity. The emphasis on statistical model building among social scientists is strong. Cesario, Simon, and Kinne (1970) rationalized this tendency as fulfilling the need to replace informed judgment with objective evaluation procedures. Yet many social scientists recognize the considerable difficulties in determining causal import estimates needed for any evaluation. Selowsky and Taylor (1971) initiated their detailed regression analysis of the rate of return to nutrition analysis with the statement that they had to "resort to statistical sleight of hand to apply theory to inadequate data." We have already questioned the underlying theory used to construct statistical models. Moreover, data availability and quantitative research techniques often lead to analyses that are probably neither adequate examinations of the theories that are proposed nor adequate bases for judging the effects of policies and programs. In this chapter we examine four aspects of research methodology in health: the ethics of research, general measurement problems, specific health data measurement problems, and regression analysis, the use of which has spread from econometrics to other social sciences.

ETHICS OF RESEARCH IN HEALTH PROBLEMS

The problem of ethics in research does not seem to enter sufficiently into most discussions of social science research, although problems may be as prevalent as they are in health research but less evident. Ethical problems of investigating the impact of a new treatment method or drug are complex. To determine if the treatment is effective, one usually establishes experimental groups, who receive the treatment, and control groups, who receive none (although they may be led to believe that they are being treated). If the treatment is effective, one may question the ethics of withholding general distribution; but if the treatment is not effective, it would be equally unethical to disperse it without adequate testing. Additionally, the large number of potential side effects makes it unlikely that any testing program will determine all potential negative impacts of a treatment that appears effective in combating a disease. There are no simple choices in investigating curative methods that would satisfy all demands of ethics.

The problem of ethics in preventive measures and nutrition programs appears somewhat more clear-cut. Some studies to determine increased productivity from disease treatment or nutrition increases seem blatantly outrageous. For example, Basta and Churchill (1974) reported that productivity improved when anemia was cured. To prove the point, some workers were not treated. Florencis and Evenson (unpublished) reported that persons who had lost substantial amounts of weight on a semistarvation diet had substantial decreases in productivity. Kraut and Muller (1946) reported that decreases in caloric consumption lowered worker productivity in Nazi Germany. It seems evident that lower-than-standard nutrition levels and infections from disease (particularly parasitic infections) will decrease productivity of individuals and reduce their ability to learn. Subsidizing social science research and withholding food from persons to prove this point is probably unnecessary, since such studies will most likely reach the same general conclusions that anyone could draw from an application of common sense to the problem. If, on the other hand, a research study were to show that malnutrition and debilitating diseases do not reduce an individual's productivity, one would have to question seriously the research techniques, the data used, or the work environment. The funds invested in this type of study would be better spent on food and health care.

However, it is not simply the fault of the researchers but, rather, of a social decision process that requires quantification of costs and benefits to justify health investments as opposed to other social investments. The main justification for this procedure is that general scientific knowledge and common sense may tell us the direction of associations between health status and economic outcomes; but in order to choose between alternative policies and programs in a world of scarce resources, we must also know the magnitude of the impact. Thus, these quantified techniques are likely to continue. We believe, however, that existing social science theories and methods have very limited chances for accurately estimating this impact. In the remainder of this chapter we discuss some of the more specific problems with data analysis and statistical models that support this view.

GENERAL MEASUREMENT PROBLEMS

There are at least four general sources of measurement problems underlying most analyses: data-gathering instruments, governmental data sources, transferability of results, and isolation of effects. Chossey, Van Veen, and Young (1967) investigated the use of questionnaires as opposed to observation in assessing food consumption patterns. They thought that the questionnaires were highly preferable, since a much larger sample could be covered and highly trained interviewers were not required. They based their conclusion upon the support that the questionnaire results gave to their preanalysis hypothesis. Nonetheless, it is quite possible that the questionnaire technique produces less accurate results, since interpretation of questions will often vary among participants. Questionnaires and observation are the two main data-gathering instruments, and both suffer from the same potential contamination of information. In field experimentation it is often quite difficult to ensure a total separation of individuals into control and experimental groups, and this increases the likelihood that either data-gathering instrument will not be sufficient for calculating the impacts of a program.

Naturally, with all data-gathering instruments, one is faced with the problem of representative sampling. Virtually no evaluation investigates an entire population. A sample is often drawn that does not meet the strict criteria for representativeness, yet the results are still generalized to the entire country.

Researchers in field experiments confront two separate problems. Governmental data sources are often generalizations of relatively representative sampling, but this data is usually generated by many different agencies. Data may be incomplete, and the assumptions used in projections and generalizations of data by different agencies may not be obvious or consistent.

The problem of generalizing results is further magnified in the transfer of information from one country to another. The gain to scientific investigation occurs when the results of experiments can be generalized to other situations. If this transfer cannot occur, there will be no knowledge base upon which to build and there will be a continuing replication of similar experiments. What worked in one country may not be transferable owing to cultural, political, social, and

FIGURE 8.1

General Data Measurement Problems

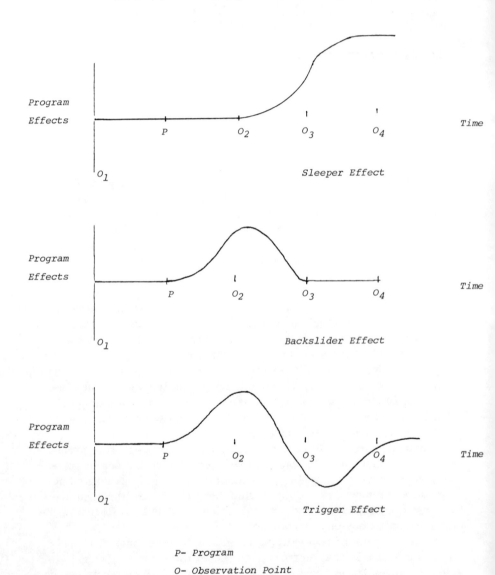

P- Program
O- Observation Point

Source: Green (1977b). Reprinted by permission.

98

economic differences among countries (Cesario, Simon, and Kinne 1970). Many times these differences will escape foreign researchers, either because of their lack of complete familiarity with the country or its values, or biases built in from their own training. Thus, health programs intended to raise nutritional standards or to create economic incentives for individual action are often based on food consumption patterns not relevant to the country in which they are developed.

Most field studies are conducted by implementing some data-gathering instrument before the program begins and at some point after it has begun, in order to determine the impacts of the program. Green (1977b) described three potential problems that would result in data analysis from observation at different points, leading to questionable results. He called these factors the "sleeper" or delayed effect, the backslider effect, and the trigger effect. These factors are summarized in Figure 8.1. The sleeper effect occurs when there is a time lag between the program and the response it elicits. This problem can also occur when there is a delay in knowledge transfer from participants to nonparticipants. The backslider effect occurs when there is some immediate change as a result of the program but reinforcement is needed to continue the program effects. The trigger effect occurs when the program induces people to take action earlier than they would have. There would be an immediate effect of the program followed by a drop below the normal level before the program implementation. Udry (1972) found this effect in a study of mass media advertising and birth control measures.

One can see from Figure 8.1 that if observations are made at 0_2, no impact will be found if the sleeper effect is operating, and a positive but short-lived impact will be found if the backslider or trigger effect is operating. It is clear that continuing observation may be needed to determine the true effectiveness of the program.

Green (1977a) pointed to another important observation problem. In tracing the relationship between effectiveness and spending levels, Green posited a threshold spending level. Spending below this level would result in no measurable effectiveness; spending above it would have increasingly higher effectiveness levels, although at potentially diminishing rates.

SPECIAL MEASUREMENT
PROBLEMS IN HEALTH PROJECTS

Principal problems in data measurement in health projects are the separation of effects between intervening variables and health-related variables, and appropriate measurements for health status problems. Similar problems, of course, exist in other social science research. For example, in measuring nutritional gains from increased consumption, researchers may find no change in general health status or work productivity if food is improperly prepared or no consideration is given to the relationship between time and frequency of meals and work activities. Therefore, intensive programs that teach the use of new foods and ensure their availability may appear to have failed if other factors are not considered. Kallen (1969) echoed a familiar problem when he called attention to the fact that the alleged association between malnutrition and intellectual development may have its origin in extraneous factors peripherally related to malnutrition. He stated that most studies of malnutrition and intellectual development involved children who were hospitalized, or from lower income groups. Hospitalization would lead to lethargy and a lack of stimulation that would hinder intellectual development. The apathy that may exist in children of lower income groups and restrict their development would not be solved simply by improving nutritional standards.

Finding appropriate ways to measure nutritional or health status can also be problematic. For example, Stine, Saratsiotis, and Furno (1967) proposed that several physical measurements be used to indicate the health status of children, since the correlations with health differ among income groups. Burk and Ezekiel (1967) discussed several methods of determining nutritional status. These included estimating food consumption in particular countries, converting this consumption into measures of available nutrition, and comparing the result with standard nutrition levels. However, they mentioned several problems with this method, including difficulty in determining nutrient content of food and the fact that the method would ignore distribution, seasonal fluctuations, and losses owing to inadequate storage, transportation, and processing. Berg and Muscat (1973) identified an additional problem in that the measurement technique ignores the effects of food preparation, distribution within the family, and health problems that reduce food absorption. As an alternative to measuring nutrition status directly, Jay (1973) and Schuftan (unpublished) suggested using a measure of household income as a proxy.

STATISTICAL MODELS—REGRESSION ANALYSIS

Regression analysis is frequently used to account for the influence of intervening variables. The basic procedure uses statistical procedures designed to calculate the coefficients, b_i's, of the following type of equation:

$$Y = b_0 + \sum_{i=1}^{n} b_i X_i \qquad (8.1)$$

where Y = measure of output,

b_0 = constant term,

b_i = coefficient for input i and represents the change in output for a unit change in input, and

X_i = amount of input i.

Statistical tests of significance are applied to the coefficients to determine if, in fact, the input has had a nonzero effect on the output. The implied assumptions involved in using a linear model such as equation 8.1 are that the effect of any input on the output is independent of the quantity of the other inputs and that each input always has the same effect on output. The validity of these assumptions is questionable. They would imply, for example, that if work productivity is the output variable and caloric consumption one of the input variables, then additional caloric consumption would have the same effect on productivity regardless of the amount of total caloric consumption. If 2,500 calories is the required amount for physical work, with no weight gain or loss, then additional caloric consumption for individuals below the standard level will probably result in some increase in productivity, whereas increased caloric consumption for individuals above the standard level may lead to decreases in productivity. This diminishing productivity of increasing levels of inputs is probably relevant for other input and output measures. Regression analysis can still be used with some other (nonlinear) functional forms that allow for diminishing marginal productivity. An oft-used model is a multiplicative function, given by:

$$Y = a_0 \prod_{i=1}^{n} X_i^{a_i} = a_0 X_1^{a_1} X_2^{a_2} X_3^{a_3} \ldots \ldots X_n^{a_n} \qquad (8.2)$$

where a_i is the output elasticity of input i (the percentage increase in output for a 1 percent increase in input i). A logarithmic transformation will convert this equation to linear form for linear regression analysis. The functional formulation chosen is an important limitation of the interpretation of results of regression analysis, since different formulation will often yield different results.

The multicollineation of input variables, the exclusion of potentially important input variables, and the use of proxies for variables for which data gathering is difficult also create significant difficulties for the reliability of regression analysis results. A main multicollinear problem in health program analysis, as in other social science analyses, is the relationship between an individual's socioeconomic status and resource availability. If one measures knowledge gain from a particular health education program, it is not easy to separate the causal effects of the health program from those attributable to the socioeconomic backgrounds of the individuals studied. For example, Chernichovsky (1977) estimated food intake as a function of income, family size, education, region of the country, and other demographic variables. All of these "independent" variables are probably related to each other, and the effect of any one of them on food intake would not be possible to isolate with regression analysis.

In the Selowsky and Taylor (1971) analysis of rate of return for infant nutrition, there are problems with multicollineation of included and excluded variables in the four-equation regression model. Here, productivity is estimated in terms of included variables, such as age, education, and IQ. But excluded variables—such as work experience, job classification, and socioeconomic status—may be just as important in explaining work productivity.

Finally, it is often difficult to obtain data for certain variables. For example, Malenbaum (1970) attempted to show the relationship between agricultural output and health. It seems clear that such output is related to the health status of specific workers. However, these data were apparently unavailable, so Malenbaum used physician-population ratios and infant mortality rates as proxies for health status. An important purpose of regression analysis is to establish causality between input variables and output. Proxy variables affect predictive capability. A significant relationship between infant mortality and agricultural output would not necessarily indicate that reductions in infant mortality would increase agricultural output. Rather, a change in the input for which infant mortality was used as a proxy could lead to improvements in agricultural output.

Regression analysis only establishes an association between output and input variables. Causality between the variables (a change in an input variable will lead to a change in the output variable) is based upon the underlying theory used to create the model. If the theory is questionable, as the controversy over different explanations for the effect of health on economic growth would indicate, it is difficult to choose between alternative explanations of the associations observed.

The existence of a number of reasonable explanations of any set of associations, combined with the problems of quantifying such theories and of statistically estimating these quantified models, all make it difficult, if not impossible, to "prove" that a particular program has a particular effect. Thus, the results achieved by evaluation of the effectiveness or benefits of alternative health (or any other) programs may not be very reliable, and they may be subject to differing interpretations. Since social science theories and methods seem to be incapable of developing clear choice criteria or measuring them, it becomes more important that decision makers understand the alternative arguments and the limitations of empirical criteria. Economic analysis can perhaps be most useful when it identifies the specific arguments, assumptions, and values behind alternative ways of evaluating systems, as we hope we have done with regard to the evaluation of health and nutrition education policy and program alternatives.

9
A CASE STUDY OF TANZANIA

co-authored with T. L. Maliyamkono and A. Ishumi

INTRODUCTION

Poor health conditions undoubtedly contribute to the relatively high infant mortality rate and low life expectancy in Tanzania. In 1972 there were 162.5 deaths per 1,000 persons under one year of age (ten times higher than most developed countries) and a life expectancy of approximately 44 years. These statistics are typical of most African nations and reflect the importance of intensive effort in health-related investments in these countries. These conditions are often attributed to a lack of sanitary and other related measures that would prevent the spread of disease. The problem is often compounded by a lack of adequate medical facilities throughout the country.

The radio campaigns established in Tanzania in the early 1970s were important steps in the direction of improving health conditions through the instruction of a large segment of the population with regard to appropriate sanitary measures (constructing and using latrines, obtaining clean drinking water, eliminating stagnant water areas, and wearing shoes) in the "Myu ni Afya" ("Man Is Health") campaign in 1973 and appropriate nutrition standards in the "Chakula ni Uhai" ("Food Is Life") campaign in 1975. However, these campaigns were of short duration—three months in the case of "Mtu ni Afya" and four months for "Chakula ni Uhai"—and have not been repeated. These two campaigns were the fourth and fifth in a series of radio campaigns that were originally oriented toward political issues (a discussion of the election of 1971) and social issues (discussions of the function of

---

This chapter was coauthored by T. L. Maliyamkono, professor of the economics of education, and A. Ishumi, professor of the sociology of education, both at the University of Dar es Salaam.

planning and of Tanzanian history and achievements since independence).

The content of these programs, particularly the "Mtu ni Afya"
campaign, which is the focus of this chapter, reflects the integration
of diverse elements in Tanzania's development. The year 1970 was
proclaimed Adult Education Year by Tanzania's president, Julius
Nyerere, and emphasized the reduction of adult illiteracy. The "Mtu
ni Afya" campaign, though aimed at health standards, was also used
to reinforce literacy training through the distribution of two 48-page
booklets to all program participants. The emphasis on widespread
education regarding the causes of disease and the relationship of poor
health conditions to the spread of disease reflects a trend toward na-
tionwide participation in development rather than a centrally controlled
effort. This is consistent with the "education for self-reliance" policy
enunciated by Nyerere.

The basic purpose of this chapter is to evaluate the impact of
the "Mtu ni Afya" campaign. There are two paths along which this
evaluation may proceed. The first reflects the literature of traditional Western economics in the evaluation of the economic impacts
of a particular action. In this methodology one compares the cost of
a particular activity with the benefits generated. This approach to
health investment evaluation was examined in more detail in Chapter
5. An alternative approach is to examine an activity in its structural
context. From this perspective, one examines an alternative in terms
of its consistency and integration with other elements of society.
This requires an investigation of Tanzania's path of development, education policies, utilization of mass media, and structure of health
care.

Different strategies are available to Tanzania for reducing its
health problems. While each of these alternatives may have similar
impacts in terms of disease reduction and, hence, the calculation of
economic benefits, the power relations in terms of which groups control the implementation of health programs may be quite different.
These other effects may have far-reaching importance for Tanzania's
development. For example, the "Mtu ni Afya" program stressed
self-help preventive measures to reduce disease incidence. This educational approach was oriented toward a decentralized, self-reliant
path. Alternative approaches might have stressed curative measures,
giving more power and authority to medical institutions and trained
persons in the country. Analysis of structural, power, and class relationships is not within the context of typical cost-benefit analysis,
which tends to be quantitatively oriented. For this reason we first
discuss other elements of Tanzanian development to place the "Mtu
ni Afya" project in its appropriate structural context, and then analyze
the project from a standard cost-benefit approach.

NATIONAL DEVELOPMENT IN TANZANIA

The past few decades have witnessed a fairly uniform development strategy on the part of many newly independent nations. This strategy has focused primary attention on the rate of capital accumulation and the utilization of advanced technologies taken from more industrialized countries. This strategy has tended to intensify the dependence of developing countries and has often led to the domination of local economies by small elites. Education development has followed a parallel path, although accumulation of human capital has been emphasized.

The specific developmental strategies of Tanzania have clearly been affected by the personality of President Nyerere and his closest advisers. Yet the hallmarks of this strategy—independence from international capital, minimization of the power of a state bureaucratic elite in favor of decentralization and mass participation, and emphasis on collective, village-based development—have their roots in the particular conditions of preindependence Tanganyika. First, Tanzania was perhaps the African state least transformed by international capitalism, and hence, had the least direct dependence on foreign investment. Consequently, it had relatively more leeway for independent development. Second, the nation lacked a strong export sector to tie it to international markets, and consequently it lacked a strong "national bourgeoisie" with both power and colonial culture. Basic market activities generally fell to Asian nationals, who engaged in trade in services. However, their minority status has minimized their political power in subsequent years. Third, the preindependence colonial administration had developed surprisingly few professional state administrators among the native population, thus minimizing entrenched local political establishments. In 1961, at the time of independence, there were fewer than 150 university graduates and only 176 students in the sixth form of secondary school.

The absence of a strongly concentrated domestic land-owning class made possible a development strategy based on community action and self-reliance without tremendous class struggles. Nevertheless, the early strategy of the national political party—the Tanganyika African National Union (TANU)—was extremely tentative in this direction, and it was at least partly the failure of the First Five-Year Plan (1965–69) to attract foreign capital that moved policy in a more innovative direction. This move was also facilitated by certain aspects of the social structure of African nationals. The widespread use of Swahili and the proliferation of tribes, none of which was effectively dominant, made for a society in which Tanzanians perceived their mutual relations as workers and peasants. Thus, the shift in policy beginning with the 1967 Arusha Declaration generated relatively little direct and overt popular opposition, despite the fact that it put extreme pressure on those with elitist tendencies.

This declaration, while consistent with the philosophy of Nyerere, came as a surprise to neighboring countries and foreign investors. De La Rue (1967) reported that nationalization was quick and reaction by British banks was strong to prevent a repetition of nationalization in other African countries, since the relation of net profit to investment rates ranged from 75 to 200 percent for these banks in developing nations.

There were five main themes in the Arusha Declaration that De La Rue (1967) felt were the basis for further Tanzanian development. These were as follows:

Self-Reliance: Development should benefit all Tanzanians and should be dependent upon Tanzanians, since other nations will put their own interests first.

Rural Development: With over 90 percent of the population living in rural areas and a surplus of rural labor and land, development must focus on rural areas rather than an urban elite.

Equity: A just society requires that differences in income levels be reduced and that the rise of an elite class—whether in the public or private sector—be prevented.

National Economic Control: To ensure self-reliance, public-cooperative and public-controlled sectors of the economy must be large in relation to the total economy.

Socialism: Socialist development must be broader than public control and include effective and widespread participation in decision making.

The policy direction initiated by the Arusha Declaration in 1967, however, was to undergo considerable intensification by the TANU Guidelines of 1971. These guidelines intensified the thrust toward decentralizing power and decision making, democratizing authority, balancing rural/urban development, and increasing "worker participation." The rationale was summed up in the TANU paper, "Decentralization."*

The purpose of both the Arusha Declaration and of Mwongozo was to give the people power over their own lives and their own development. We have made great progress in seizing power from the hands of the capitalists and the traditionalists, but we must face the fact that, to the mass of the peo-

_____

*Dar es Salaam, 1972.

ple, power is still something wielded by others—even if
on their behalf.

Thus it has gradually become obvious that, in order to
make a reality of our policies of socialism and self-reliance, the planning and control of development in this
country must be exercised at the local level to a much
greater extent than at present. . . . These proposals in
fact follow logically from the Arusha Declaration and from
Mwongozo, and from the basic principles of Ujamaa. For
they imply putting trust in the people. And if we cannot do
that, we have no claim to be socialists.

Mwongozo considerably strengthened the position of workers and
peasants and, indeed, is responsible for a heightened intensity of
worker struggles and democratic participation from below. Yet the
humanism of Nyerere and the paternalism of some of the leaders are
not alone responsible for this shift. As Shivji (1975) noted, Mwongozo
occurred shortly after the overthrow of similarly progressive regimes
in Guinea and Uganda, essentially by petty bourgeois forces. Fearing
comparable developments at home, the elite in the public sector may
have chosen the admittedly precarious strategy of extending its mass
base at the expense of the middle and lower levels of the petty bourgeoisie.

Thus, the policies initiated in 1971 brought about a substantive
shift in power and consciousness of peasants and workers, which has
not yet run its course. The struggle can be expected to continue for
some time along these newly developed lines. The implications for
education in Tanzania are extensive and will be discussed below.

AN OVERVIEW OF EDUCATION REFORMS

There are four education reforms (discussed in more detail in
Maliyamkono [1977]) that relate to the various changes in development
policy in Tanzania. The first reform, covering the period from independence in 1961 to about 1966, was the integration of curriculum.
Reflecting the overall strategy of nationalism rather than tribalism
and unity rather than division based on ethnic, racial, and regional
differences, this policy had several goals: the removal of the racial
system of education promulgated by the colonial government, the establishment of local educational authorities, and the unification of
teacher education. The policies of the reform were the vast expansion of primary education, the standardization of curriculum and examinations, and the gradual elimination of school fees. Owing to
early TANU anticolonialist orientation, it also involved the elimination

of agricultural education, which had been reserved in colonial days for the "inferior" Africans, and the universalization of instruction in English, which had been restricted in the system of colonial education.

The shortcomings of this reform soon became evident and indeed mirrored the general problems in the early TANU strategy. The growth of primary education by the removal of school entrance blocks and by reductions in the drop-out rate, though progressive, added to the problem of unemployment among graduates. The emphasis on Western urban culture (symbolized by the use of English) reinforced negative attitudes toward rural development and heavy migration to urban areas. Moreover, the educational pyramid remained about as steep as before, and the reform had little effect on the degrees of economic inequality.

The second major reform, the expansion of secondary and university education for manpower requirements in the 1960s, was a logical extension of early TANU developmental policy and a response to some of the shortcomings mentioned in the earlier educational reform strategy. Manpower requirement programs were prompted by the labor vacuum caused by departing expatriate personnel and the general growth of labor demand as a result of favorable economic conditions in the 1960s.

As some of the major obstacles to entry into primary school were eliminated, the number of graduates increased to such an extent that it became a national problem. Private endeavors (especially by missionaries) to open private secondary schools and homecraft centers did not solve the problem, which was aggravated by the shift of labor demand from primary to secondary graduates. Worse still, primary school graduates with a mean age of 14 were too young to enter direct employment. The curriculum of primary school education was incomplete in the sense that pupils were prepared to enter secondary education and not to return to the land. One could argue, therefore, that primary education became increasingly expensive, considering direct expenditures and the negligible effects on skills within the labor pool.

Some of the goals of the pre-1967 reform were achieved. There was a rapid expansion in the number of qualified personnel, and the educational pyramid became considerably less steep. But in addition to the increased unemployment among secondary school graduates, the reform exacerbated the urban/rural imbalance, promoted excess migration to urban areas, and had little effect on relative salaries or other forms of economic inequality.

The spotty successes of these two educational reform efforts again paralleled the tradition-bound commitments of early Tanzanian development policy. While some aspects of faltering educational policy in this period were doubtless attributable to the young nation's lack of experience in social planning and the state of administrative institutions, there were basic structural forces at work as well. These seem related to Tanzania's adoption, under the leadership of a petty bourgeoisie emerging confidently from independence struggles, of a traditional capitalist developmental strategy in which high profits, reinvestment of private gain, and the maximization of capital growth held the center stage. Thus, educational policy was devoted exclusively to the development of labor skills required by the traditional model that was pushed by the government leadership.

The year 1967 saw a major and fundamental revision of social goals in Tanzania with the Arusha Declaration. This declaration became the official party and government basis for all policies, including those on education. President Nyerere subsequently released the pamphlet "Education for Self-Reliance," which has become the basis for all major educational changes since that time. "Education for Self-Reliance" (ESR) was intended to change the attitudes of the elite, to make education relevant and practical, and to make the school a part of the communal economic enterprise.

The goal of self-reliance affected education in several ways. First, the emphasis on academic subjects was lessened, in favor of such practical concerns as health and nutrition. Second, the schools were to favor cooperative rather than competitive relations among students, and education was to relate closely to community activities and needs. Third, the primary schools substituted Swahili for English and began to eliminate colonial aspects of the school curriculum. Fourth, the primary school curriculum was to be complete in itself and not a preparation for secondary education. Fifth, primary education was to be made relevant to rural development, since the majority of graduates would engage in agricultural activities.

In terms of concrete and immediate social and economic results, ESR has not proven a great success. There have been some changes in the distribution of income, economic opportunity, and rural/urban migration, but it is unlikely that ESR was responsible for more than small increments of the progress made. Rather, the reform must be judged on its contribution to the foundations of Tanzanian socialism and self-reliance.

In these larger terms, the ESR reform must be seen as partially successful, its limitations being a reflection of the necessarily comprehensive nature of social change and the contradictions of recent TANU strategy. While educational reform has contributed to the creation of socialist consciousness and collective solidarity, the programs have been hindered by the negative attitude of school administrators and teachers adhering to the old traditions. More fundamentally, the slowness of program development reflects the still powerful opposition of educated political and social elites, to whom the new development strategy poses a threat.

The last major reform, decentralization of education, closely parallels the deepening commitment to self-reliance and participatory democracy embodied in the Mwongozo resolutions of 1971. The goal of this reform was to increase participation on the local village level, further undercutting the power of administrative elites. The expansion of adult literacy also had this end.

Perhaps it is too early to evaluate most of these educational reforms, since reform—unlike political revolution—is a slow process. Another problem lies in the difficulty of evaluation, because the parameters are not as discrete as outputs of a production industry. What is advocated is a growing awareness of education as one of the tools for improving community services.

The ESR reform was particularly important to adult education, since policies enunciated in the Arusha Declaration in 1967 eventually led to the declaration of 1970 as Adult Education Year. A massive adult literacy program was begun, as well as the adult-oriented radio programs of which "Mtu ni Afya" was a part. The change in approach to adult education is reflected in the orientation of the radio program. Hall (1975) provided a brief summary of the major elements of the shift in approach. The primary features of the pre-Arusha Declaration period were paternalistic and elitist. Much of adult education was oriented in the same manner as continuing education, with an emphasis on courses designed for middle- to high-skilled persons who had completed at least primary education. That education, which was directed toward the masses, emphasized a willingness to change and a dependence on "experts" for solutions.

In the post-1970 period, the emphasis shifted from continuing formal education to education for those who had had no formal schooling, and greater attention was given to rural development needs. An attempt was also made to emphasize participation in development. The shift from a paternalistic to a participatory program is subtle, since the major problem identified in both mass education approaches is the lack of previous education for most of the people.

The Mtu ni Afya campaign may be considered paternalistic, but the primary emphasis was on education of rural adults concerning causes of disease and improvements in health practices. Additionally, the program was used to provide a practical reinforcement for the literacy campaign through the distribution of booklets.

THE ROLE OF MASS MEDIA

The overall assumption of mass media use—not only in Tanzania but everywhere in the world—is that information from a single source can flow easily and quickly to large portions of the population. Radio, newspapers, information bulletins, and (in richer countries) television serve to broadcast information to the widest possible audience.

By nature and function, mass media are educational, for they involve two parties: a source from which "new" information, solicitation, directives, and the like flow to a target population who receive this information and—presumably—respond to it. The source of information is usually seen as a center of innovation, while the intended destination of the information is the target area or target population. As informational and/or consciousness-raising devices, mass media are useful educational instruments. This explains why they are increasingly used as an educational strategy in national development, especially among the less industrialized countries. A number of community development and general self-improvement projects have increasingly drawn on the effective use of mass media, along with the conscious drive in mass literacy training.

In Tanzania, owing to the remoteness and physical inaccessibility of many of the rural communities, the shortage of necessary and sufficient manpower, and the conscious need to reinforce and perpetuate initial efforts, mass media that can reach a wider spectrum of the population in a relatively short time are increasingly used for educational purposes. The publication of more regular newspapers enjoying wider circulation, the distribution of information bulletins and agricultural manuals, and the extension of radio broadcasting time and the launching of radio programs in health care, agriculture, civics, and the like are oriented toward improving conditions in rural areas.

Supported by mass circulation papers, bulletins, and manuals, the national radio broadcasting station centered in Dar es Salaam has been a vital instrument in launching mass education campaigns in literacy, civics, health, agriculture, and nutrition. If achievements are examined, one can see that radio instruction and discussion can be a vital component of strategies in adult and general mass education.

The specific objective of radio-transmitted programs for adults is fourfold:

1. It is _motivational_. The programs stimulate adult participation in the literacy process by creating public awareness and interest and by encouraging enrollment at adult education centers.

2. It is _instructional_. The programs reinforce basic skills by providing instructions to supplement that given in the field by tutors and coordinators of various adult studies in regions throughout the country. The radio organizes "model" discussion groups and forums in which application of certain key ideas and skills is given emphasis.

3. It is _functional_. The programs stress the importance of literacy and other functional (work- and life-oriented) skills. They also stimulate public interest in rural library facilities, newspapers, information bulletins, and agricultural and other productive manuals.

4. It is <u>communicational</u> and <u>informational</u>. Centrally organized radio programs cut down communication barriers, which are formidable in a large and diverse rural area. Such programs make for a coordinated approach to development by creating a "central" information system that provides feedback on the various projects in the country. The field reports, interviews, and discussions that are broadcast reach a great many people instantaneously. Without a central broadcasting system, the communication of information and the innovations it makes possible would be hard to achieve. "Output" expectations of increased adult enrollment and attendance at adult education centers, improved efficiency and functional abilities, faster diffusion of innovations, widened scope of environmental awareness and knowledge, and general attitudinal change have all been assisted by these radio study programs.

The series of radio programs of which "Mtu ni Afya" is a part was based on earlier Tanzanian experience with radio forums in the mid-1960s and on radio forum experiences in many other countries, including India (Mathur and Neurath 1959), Canada (Nicol, et al. 1954), and Ghana (Abell 1968). These are described in more detail in Wells (1976), Hall and Dodds (1977), and Hall (1977). We draw on the latter two sources for a brief description of earlier Tanzanian experience.

The essential element in most radio forums has been the establishment of organized listening groups at the village level. The groups are typically led by a person who has received some training and who serves as a liaison between participants and central planning groups and as a discussion leader for group decision making based upon the radio lessons. Frequently, the radio broadcasts are supplemented by printed materials. Radio forums began separately in two locations in Tanzania. In 1964 a Cooperative Education Center was founded in Moshi to meet local education needs of cooperative society. Since many participants were not literate, it was found that the most useful format was to organize groups who were read to by a literate member and to supplement the discussion with radio broadcasts.

Simultaneously, in 1964 the Institute of Adult Education (IAE) of the University of Dar es Salaam, established 15 experimental groups from recently established local adult education associations in Mbeya. These groups were given instruction in English, civics, and agriculture, and served as an experimental point for IAE work on the radio campaigns.

The mass communication strategy that was initiated in 1969 set in operation six principal radio programs aimed at achieving specific goals. This specificity of objectives led to a defined program termination date. The six sequential programs are:

1. "Kupanga ni Kuchagua" (literally, "To Plan Is to Choose"), primarily aimed at educating the people on the objectives and expectations of the Second Five-Year Development Plan (1968-74).

2. "Uchaguzi ni Wako" (literally, "The Election Is Yours"), meant to educate and prepare the public for the general elections of 1971.

3. "Wakati wa Furaha" (literally, "A Time of Rejoicing"), a program designed to coincide with the country's tenth anniversary (December 1971), by providing instruction in the history of Tanzania and the achievements made since independence.

4. "Mtu ni Afya" (literally, "Man Is Health"), a health education campaign designed to urge the rural population to exercise proper health habits and sanitation and to provide basic information on disease, disease control, and the relationship between environment and disease.

5. "Chakula ni Uhai" (literally, "Food Is Life"), a nutrition campaign.

6. "Mwalimu wa Walimu" (literally, "Tutor of Tutors"), a course in the principles of adult education.

Characteristics of the first five programs are summarized in Table 9.1.

THE STRUCTURE OF HEALTH CARE

The role and structure of medical care in Tanzania are considerably influenced by government policy regarding development and provision of medical services. This is part of the country's overall policy of social development.

Because the country is vast and the population scattered, it was impossible to provide full-fledged hospitals accessible to all the widely distributed population. Consequently, a policy of "little and often" rather than "big but rare" has been adopted with regard to distribution of medical services. A great many smaller-unit services—dispensaries and rural health centers—accessible to large numbers of people have been established rather than large elegant hospitals that cannot be reached with ease. The resulting structure of facilities is pyramidal: the dispensaries, rooted in the rural countryside, form the base; there are a few hospitals at district and regional levels; and, largest but fewest, the consultant hospitals stand at the apex of the medical service delivery system (see Figure 9.1).

The smallest medical units are the rural dispensaries—formerly run by the area's local authority, and now, since the abolition of local governments in 1972, by the central government. The dispensaries are headed by a rural medical aide, although in the case of a few more

TABLE 9.1

Mass Adult Education Radio Study Campaigns

Study Program	Year	Period of Preparation	Publicity Media	Target Population	Duration (in months)	Broadcast Time	Government Expenditure on Program (Tanzanian shillings)	Number of Trained Leaders
Development Plan, "Kupanga ni Kuchagua" ("To Plan Is to Choose")	1969	Six months (1969)	Press releases; radio announcements; meetings	750	1.5	30 minutes; one per week	Not available	30-35
General Election, "Uchaguzi ni Wako" ("The Election Is Yours")	1970	Six months to one year	Press releases; radio announcements; meetings	2,250	1.0	30 minutes; one per week	Not available	150
Anniversary, "Wakati wa Furaha" ("A Time of Rejoicing")	1971	One year (1970/71)	Radio announcements; press releases; government circulars; meetings	22,500	2.5	30 minutes; one per week	81,634.95	1,854
Health, "Mtu ni Afya" ("Man Is Health")	1973	One year (1972/73)	Radio announcements; press releases; prime minister's circulars; posters; textile prints; songs; and the like	1 million	3.0	30 minutes; one per week with one repetition	1,502,000.00	75,000
Nutrition, "Chakula ni Uhai" ("Food Is Life")	1975	One year (1974/75)	Radio announcements; press releases; prime minister's circulars; posters; textile prints; songs; and the like	2 million	4.0	15 minutes; one per week with one repetition	2,500,000.00	100,000

advanced dispensaries, a medical assistant is in charge. In 1968 there were 937 rural dispensaries, 399 of which were classified as Grade A, the rest as Grade B. In 1978 there were well over 1,000 rural dispensaries.

Above these rural dispensaries are rural health centers, which are major dispensaries and serve as nuclei for anything from three to five smaller dispensaries. They are usually manned by either an assistant medical officer or a medical assistant, two nurses or midwives, two village midwives, two or three nursing orderlies, and two or three subordinate staff. A senior or junior health assistant is usually attached to the center. In 1968 there were 30 rural health centers; by the end of the Second Five-Year Plan in 1974 there were 83. The health centers had cost about $2,200 each and the equipment had been mostly provided by the United Nations International Children's Emergency Fund.

Hospitals are the next higher stage after rural health centers, staffed by doctors, trained nursing staff, supporting (technical) staff, as well as lower subordinate staff. Regional hospitals tend to be su-

FIGURE 9.1

Structure of Public Medical Facilities

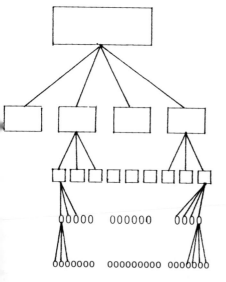

National Consustant Hospitals
1 Govt (Bugando at Mwanza)
1 Vol. Agency (KCMC at Moshi)
1 Parastatal (Muh. Med. Ctr., Dsm.)

Regional Hospitals

District Hospitals

Rural Health Centers (serving 8,000-10,000 families, i.e., c.50,000 people each)

Rural Dispensaries (serving about 1,500 families each)

perior to district hospitals; in the past, at least, a district hospital would be manned or headed by licensed (usually up-graded) medical practitioners, whereas the regional hospital was manned by registered practitioners (professionally trained and qualified personnel). Higher above these district and regional hospitals are the consultative hospitals, which handle difficult and referral cases from the lower regional hospitals and form the core of innovative and laboratory research work for the country and the wider professional world.

As a step to relieve the pressure of outpatient and dispensary work, especially in urban hospitals, health centers and clinics were planned to be built (and most have been opened) in several towns, namely Arusha, Dar es Salaam, Ifakara, Iringa, Kigoma, Morogoro, Moshi, Ntwara, and Tanga.

Gish (1973) reported that the plan was to increase the number of rural health centers from 100 to 300 and dispensaries from 110 to 2,000. The major goal was to have some medical facility within a two-hour walking distance of any person. The trend toward more rural health centers was supported by a simple analysis by Gish (1973). He compared the service possibilities from similar expenditures for one regional hospital and six rural health centers. He estimated that for a capital cost of TSh6 million* and an operating cost of TSh2 million, a regional hospital could handle 9,000 inpatient admissions, 400,000 outpatient visits, and serve a population of 10,000 to 30,000, whereas the same expenditures for rural health centers would serve a population of 30,000 to 50,000 and allow for 15,000 inpatient admissions and 1 million outpatient visits.

The past tendency to concentrate health expenditures on both hospitals and urban areas is changing. Gish (1973) reported that in 1970/71 and 1971/72, 50 percent of the capital budget went to hospitals and two-thirds of this amount was spent in the Dar es Salaam area. In 1973/74 only 15 percent of the capital budget was allocated to hospitals and only one-tenth of this amount was spent in Dar es Salaam. However, Sorkin (1976) reported that per capita health expenditures were nine times higher in Dar es Salaam than the rest of the country and four times higher in towns than rural areas. This allocation probably took place prior to the reorientation in 1973/74.

The magnitude of the shift from a centralized, urban, curative medical system to a decentralized, rural, preventive one is most clearly seen in the data presented in Table 3.2. Capital expenditures for preventive services increased from 1 percent of a total budget of $2.76 million in 1970/71 to 21 percent of a $12.22 million budget in 1976/77. Recurrent spending for preventive measures also involved

---

*Tanzanian shillings; TSh8 = U.S.$1.

substantial increases in this seven-year period. Furthermore, while capital and recurrent spending on hospitals increased during this period a greater budget allocation was made to rural health centers and dispensaries.

Since the Second Five-Year Plan, there has also been a shift in emphasis from curative to preventive measures. These include the following:

1. Better nutrition, especially for children. Since malnutrition is often the cause for the sickness and eventual death of many children in Tanzania, the Ministry of Health has been organizing teams to visit villages, towns, health centers, and clinics to give advice on how to improve diets and nutrition in general. Other ministries, especially Agriculture, have joined in advising on food-crop production.

2. Sanitation. This has centered mainly on providing funds to construct and expand durable clean water supplies, especially in rural areas. Other measures have included help in setting up viable refuse disposal systems, building latrines, and deploying garbage bins.

3. Better care for mothers and children (ante- and postnatal care). Mostly, this has consisted of advice to mothers, which has helped to check the rate of natal and child mortality. Free family planning services are provided as well.

4. Control and vaccination against communicable diseases. The government, with the cooperation of voluntary agencies, particularly the missions, has set up a unit within the Ministry of Health to further control such diseases as tuberculosis, leprosy, smallpox, and sleeping sickness.

5. Mass health education. Aimed at reinforcing the practical field measures taken, the health education program has focused on the importance and advantages of environmental cleanliness, principles of good living, principles and characteristics of good health and sanitation, dangers of epidemic diseases, ways of prevention, and the like.

"Mtu ni Afya," the mass media health education campaign launched in May 1973, has thus to be understood in the context of the changing public health policy with a growing emphasis on prevention rather than curative medicine. The potential success of the budgetary allocations and the radio programs may be seen in the data in Table 9.2, which show a general decline in disease incidence.

THE "MTU NI AFYA" CAMPAIGN

The "Mtu ni Afya" ("Man Is Health") campaign had its major focus on some 750,000 of the rural population living in rural ujamaa

TABLE 9.2

Outpatient Cases of Common Diseases

Hospital	Dysentery 1970	Dysentery 1976	Malaria 1970	Malaria 1976	Kwashiorkor 1970	Kwashiorkor 1976	Marasmus 1970	Marasmus 1976	Hookworm 1970	Hookworm 1976
1. Berega (Morogoro)	58	52	1,548	864	4	32	115	—	325	99
2. Bulongwa (Iringa)	3	25	290	350	6	21	6	5	23	30
3. Ifakara (Norogoro)	316	40	5,762	720	4,534	71	—	5	3,414	340
4. Idonda (Iringa)	51	32	—	536	232	8	—	—	31	42
5. Ilembura (Iringa)	25	10	945	784	38	37	13	14	167	23
6. Itete (Mbeya)	9	—	4,778	874	28	4	2	2	92	83
7. Kagondo (West Lake)	—	24	671	366	15	27	—	3	668	577
8. Kibosho (Moshi)	661	1,702	180	366	58	721	—	864	1,128	2,533
9. Kola-Ndoto (Shinyanga)	105	91	675	277	55	77	6	11	195	167
10. Lugala (Morogoro)	210	41	1,561	670	5	125	—	34	1,051	873
11. Lugarawa (Iringa)	202	283	902	454	122	5	3	—	80	259
12. Makiungu (Singida)	68	341	251	682	65	33	29	47	245	859
13. Mbozi (Mbeya)	39	190	210	2,070	10	219	5	145	42	418
14. Murgawanza (West Lake)	18	113	—	2,920	150	86	—	—	405	229
15. Ndolage (West Lake)	36	136	—	981	68	10	11	4	247	716
16. Nyangao (Lindi)	108	295	3,600	8,793	36	119	2	58	304	785
17. Rulenge (West Lake)	11	303	4,549	2,701	59	9	4	4	816	723
18. Utete (Coast)	244	42	5,361	854	194	64	125	12	5,383	663
Total	2,174	3,720	31,515	25,202	5,449	1,666	321	1,208	14,616	9,419

Source: Ministry of Health. Reprinted by permission.

(cooperative) villages and some 250,000 in six districts that had by that time spearheaded the national adult literacy campaign. The rationale for the focus on ujamaa villages was that, being relatively more compact than the other more scattered rural communities, they were more exposed to the dangers of communicable diseases and would therefore find the program most useful. Although the inclusion of the six districts in the target population was based on their headstart advantage in the 1971 national literacy campaign, the underlying assumption was that, with a certain amount of attainment in the knowledge of reading and writing, the population in these districts would be able to deal more effectively with the literature accompanying the radio broadcasts. Furthermore, the campaign literature would serve to reinforce reading skills.

The principal objective of this campaign was to promote preventive education, to excite and heighten in the people an awareness of their environment that would lead to reduction—if not eradication—of common diseases such as malaria, dysentery, bilharzia (schistosomiasis), and tuberculosis, which are not only responsible for the personal weakness and eventual death of many people but are also partly the cause of the vicious circle of poverty and underdevelopment in the rural areas: Disease → Poor Health → Little Productivity → Poor/Less Food (and other goods) → Disease (and Poverty). It was believed that this circle could be broken if people were given knowledge of the causes of these diseases, their symptoms, and ways of preventing or curing them at an early stage. A concomitant objective of the campaign was to encourage retention of newly acquired reading and writing skills by providing suitable reading follow-up materials to those who had participated in the national literacy drive (and asking them, when possible, to write a few things down in their notebooks).

A significant amount of prebroadcast planning was necessary for the program. This planning extended over a period of six to eight months and included writing, editing, printing, and distributing study guides and group leader manuals; writing and recording radio programs; planning and running training seminars; and publicizing the campaign.

Several national organizations were involved in planning and implementing the project. Hall (1977) listed the following ministries with their responsibilities, as stated at the conclusion of the project:

National Ministry of Health, Health Education Unit

Content ot textbooks and radio programs.
Production of radio programs.
Assistance from health education personnel in recruiting, training, distribution, and supervision.

Ministry of National Education, Adult Education Directorate

Overall organization of recruitment of group members and leaders, distribution of materials to groups, training of group leaders, and supervision.
Assistance in editing textbooks.

Prime Minister's Office, Rural Development Division

Administrative support for regional and district development directors (senior administrative officers of the decentralized government).
Provision of training facilities (rural training centers).
Assistance in training.

Radio Tanzania

Assistance in editing radio programs.
Provision of free air time.

Tanganyika African National Union (TANU)

Overall mobilization and recruitment of group members and leaders.
Assistance in training.

Institute of Adult Education (IAE)

Day-to-day campaign coordination.
Editing and production of textbooks.
Drafting, editing, and production of group leaders' manual.
Development of training methods and materials.
Coordination of publicity.
Production of posters.
Evaluation.

The program, which lasted for 12 weeks (May 14 to August 15, 1973) consisted of 12 separate programs of 30-minute duration. Each of these programs was broadcast twice during its scheduled week. The dates were chosen to avoid major planting or harvesting times. The program developed six main themes through lessons, presentations, and group discussion. The six themes and their corresponding durations were: (1) malaria, three weeks; (2) water, two weeks; (3) dysentery, two weeks; (4) hookworm, two weeks; (5) bilharzia, one week; and (6) tuberculosis, two weeks.

Each group study meeting was synchronized with a relevant radio program. While the radio program had as far as possible been recorded in the field with villagers themselves talking about real problems and experiences, the study meeting was to provide a complementary "real-life situation" in which people discussed common health hazards and ways of preventing or combating disease. Thus, for any particular week or day in the week, the radio broadcast and the study meeting in the field were to support and reinforce each other.

The typical sequence of activity during class time was as follows:

1. The class would gather while the radio played songs and poems related to the campaign and made short announcements concerning the general program (ten minutes of programming time).

2. The group would listen for 20 minutes to the formal radio program (presentation of lesson).

3. After the broadcast, the group leader or some competent person appointed from among the group members would read aloud the appropriate section or passage in the textbook.

4. After reading aloud, group discussion would begin, centering on the relevance of the material presented.

5. If the information presented for the day seemed important and/or provoking, the group would make definite resolutions as to what they could do—as individuals or as a group, at the center or in the community—to prevent the disease in question.

6. After the group meeting—during the week between class times—the members would put these resolutions into effect either in their own homes (such as cleaning up household containers) or in a group project (such as clearing the bush near their adult class center).

With regard to the diseases under study (malaria, dysentery, hookworm, bilharzia, and tuberculosis), the main theme was broken down into lesson/discussion units, which highlighted:

The disease and its danger to man,
Manifestations of the disease (its environment),
Symptoms of the disease in man (its identification) and how the disease spreads, and
Ways of combating the disease (prevention and/or cure).

Making lessons for adult learners effective had important implications for the preparation and training of teachers or group leaders and also for the preparation of teaching aids.

Altogether, 75,000 group leaders were trained, through 2,000 divisional seminars, to lead group study discussions intended to involve 1 million adult learners. The training of group leaders for the

"Mtu ni Afya" campaign was constructed in stages for national, zonal, district, division, and ward levels. It was expected that those who attended training at a higher level would train others at the subsequent stage.

At the national level, a two-day briefing seminar, which was held at the Institute of Adult Education (IAE) in Dar es Salaam, was attended by about 30 participants from central and regional educational and health institutions—from the IAE, the Cooperative Education Center in Moshi, the TANU, the Women's Organization, the Prime Minister's Office, the National Service, and the prison and police force. The participants at this seminar were acquainted with the history of the campaign—its origin, purpose, and organization. They were also taught methods of conducting and organizing subsequent training seminars in their respective zonal areas.

More articulate and detailed training work was done at the zonal level, where participants were expected to serve as tutors for the subsequent district seminars. Thus, participants at the zonal seminars were briefed on both methods of conducting similar seminars and methods of study at the subsequent district level. A total of 240 individuals from the Institute of Adult Education offices in Dar es Salaam and the regions, the literacy teacher training teams, the Ministry of Health, and the Cooperative College were trained at the zonal seminars; they, in turn, were to be engaged in training others at the district level.

Training seminars at the district level—and, subsequently, at the divisional or ward levels—were much more elaborate, since they involved individuals who would be in much closer contact with the adult study groups in the field. Training was focused on organizational methods for group study, in which the adult learners would be engaged. It was also aimed at equipping the participants with the skills for organizing the anticipated 2,000 seminars at the lower divisional (ward) level.

Thus, 240 officials had been trained at zonal seminars, who in turn trained over 3,000 participants at about 65 district seminars, who finally trained the 75,000 group leaders and advisers at 2,000 different divisional seminars. Teaching aids at the seminars included books, cassette-taped copies of sample programs, seminar timetables, group leaders' manuals, and a 16-page flip-over, which had been prepared with key notes on the group study method and campaign theme.

The approach taken for the "Mtu ni Afya" campaign emphasized practical activity both as a learning experience in itself and as an act of self-improvement and/or environmental improvement. During the training of the group leaders, the goal was stressed to have each group respond to the health campaign with some physical evidence of environmental change.

It was hoped that in the course of group discussions after the formal radio presentation, members of the group might decide to undertake some project that would reinforce what they had learned and simultaneously improve their environment and prevent disease. This stress on practical action colored not only the verbal discussion in the course of training but also the suggestions of projects in the Group Leader's Manual.

As indicated elsewhere, the population target for the "mtu ni Afya" campaign was 1 million—the figure upon which the number of teaching-learning materials and other considerations had been based. However, the actual figure of the people who registered ("turned up") for classes was a little more than 2 million, 52 percent men and 48 percent women. About 50 percent of the participants were between the ages of 20 and 40, while 18 percent were less than 20 and 25 percent were above 40 years of age (Institute of Adult Education 1974).

Of the total number of adults who registered for the "Mtu ni Afya" classes, 22 percent had had no formal education at all, while 37 percent had some measure of literacy though no precise formal educational attainment; 29 percent of the population had attended, though not necessarily completed, grade school (standards one through eight). Very few participants (0.5 percent) had acquired secondary school education.

The overwhelming majority of the attendants (93 percent) identified themselves as farmers—a fact that is probably not surprising when it is understood that between 93 and 95 percent of the country's population live in the rural areas, where the main subsistence occupation is agriculture.

Groups ranged in size from two persons to several hundred, with an average group size of 18 members. The typical group size was 25 to 30, double the "ideal" size of 15. In fact, attendance was nearly twice what was expected.

While most groups (73 percent) met for the Monday broadcast, a full 9 percent met on days other than those on which radio broadcasts were made (18 percent met on Wednesdays). It is therefore likely that over 10 percent of the 75,000 did not utilize the radio at all.

Although 2 million people registered for the course, only 77 percent appeared the first day. With a fairly moderate drop-out rate (compared with other adult education classes in Tanzania), the overall attendance rate was 63 percent, with only 55 percent attending in non-radio areas. (Data were not available regarding that portion of the country that did not receive a radio signal.)

EVALUATION

Essentially, there are two ways of analyzing the "Mtu ni Afya" campaign. The first is the predominantly quantitative approach of traditional Western economics. The second is a more qualitative approach analyzing the structural context in which the campaign was formulated and implemented. As one can see, the campaign was consistent with the basic tendency of national development policies (decentralization and self-reliance), national education policies (stress on adult education) and national health policies (a movement toward preventive rather than curative approaches). Clearly, the project was initiated, planned, and controlled by the central government. However, since the goal was to initiate local involvement, central control of the project is not inconsistent with the trend of national policy toward decentralization.

Consistency with other elements of development or government policy is a necessary but not sufficient condition for determining whether or not a particular investment was worthwhile. Any society operates with scarce resources and must make choices among alternative uses of those resources so that the "best" results may be achieved. It is the definition of the word best that causes so much controversy over project evaluation and has led Western economists to rely so heavily on the economic tools of cost, cost-effectiveness, and cost-benefit analysis.

The post-"Mtu-ni-Afya"-campaign field investigation we undertook for cost, cost-effectiveness, and cost-benefit analysis had two main objectives. The first was to evaluate the long-term effectiveness of the campaign in terms of its original goals. A principal goal had been to promote preventive education among the rural population and to heighten its sensitivity to environmental hazards. We wanted to evaluate the extent to which the program had succeeded—four and a half years after its formal operation—in affecting people's attitudes and skills in dealing with disease prevention.

The second allied objective of the study was to gauge the cost of the program in terms of the human, financial, and material resource inputs and to assess the viability of the program against the outputs and, more particularly, against the effectiveness and the benefits of the campaign.

For the first objective of the study, the researchers chose the questionnaire technique as the most appropriate instrument, especially with respect to gauging changes and/or adaptations in people's attitudes and beliefs. It is understandable that, for the most part, attitudes and beliefs will influence actions and choices. Responses to questionnaire items would then serve as indicators of the respondent's real disposition and, indirectly, as indicators of the change or lack of change in attitude and practice, which could, in turn, be taken to be a function of the "Mtu ni Afya" educational campaign. While the questionnaire was the primary data source, it was combined with observation of the domestic surroundings of the subjects. The questionnaire was administered to 2,500 persons in ten districts.

For the second objective of assessing the progam's costs and benefits, the researchers relied much on interviews with officials in relevant government ministries and parastatal institutions, who were closely connected with the various radio campaigns, and with physicians. Interviews were conducted with key or knowledgeable officials in the Ministries of Health, Education, and Agriculture; the Institute of Adult Education; and the national broadcasting unit (Radio Tanzania). From these interviews it was learned that it is difficult—perhaps impossible at this time—to arrive at a comprehensive figure for the costs of the program. This is because not every input was centrally administered or paid for: There was multiplicity and overlap of institutions and also a large measure of volunteer work rendered by various institutions and private individuals, at various levels of operation. Physicians were interviewed for their estimates of potential benefits in terms of reduction of disease attendant on changes in health practices.

This study was conducted as a small follow-up to the somewhat larger study conducted during and at the conclusion of the campaign and reported in substantial detail in Hall (1977). Several limitations were encountered in conducting a study four years after the campaign terminated. The major limitation was the inability to uncover completely the total project costs. Many agencies and institutions in Tanzania participated in the campaign, and their contributions are not included as project costs in any of the earlier documentations of the campaign. We therefore rely on Hall's report of project costs, which mostly cover direct campaign preparation, and we impute values for radio and participant time. The radio station is government-operated and used primarily for adult education programs. Thus, it may be argued that the "Mtu ni Afya" campaign, since it is an adult education program, should not be assessed costs for radio time. Yet alternative uses of the radio time were possible, and some assigned cost to represent the opportunity cost of the radio time is appropriate. An additional limitation of this study is that it must rely on people's memories rather than immediate responses. It is important, nonetheless, since it provides information concerning long-term effects of the campaign measured in terms of continued practice of better health standards and recall of health knowledge.

There are no really adequate a priori hypotheses applicable to the results of the current study. For example, if it had been found that 40 percent of the participants had changed their health practices immediately following the campaign, it would be difficult to predict whether the number would decrease or increase after four years. The termination of the program and the lack of continued government interest might result in a decrease in health standards. However, diffusion of innovation theories (see Rogers and Shoemaker 1971) would lead us to predict an increase in health practices since those who adopted the changes might influence others after the campaign was terminated.

Our analysis of costs and benefits is only indicative of the application of this technique to a health campaign. It was difficult to obtain information for all the diseases and it was necessary to rely on the professional judgment of physicians regarding the connection between health practices and reduction of disease. Physicians were also able to provide information regarding duration of disease with and without treatment and death rates from disease. They did not give any indication of potential differences in work productivity. A more complete study would make use of health statistics regarding disease incidence before and after the campaign and would also include an investigation of changes in work productivity. However, this information is not currently available and one would not be able to attribute all changes in disease incidence to the "Mtu ni Afya" program. Owing to the inherent data problems, the analyses discussed below should be viewed as examples of techniques rather than reliable calculations of the program's impacts.

Cost Analysis

A complete cost analysis would require a detailed listing of all resources used in preparing and conducting the project. However, detailed record keeping was not maintained. Only expenditures for some of the explicit program activities are available from other reports of the "Mtu ni Afya" campaign (mainly Hall [1977], with which we are comparing our results). The activities for which cost information is available include: training of group leaders, production of printed material and radio programs, publicity, research, and post-campaign publications. The activities listed above were externally financed. Many other contributions to the program, particularly personnel of a variety of Tanzanian agencies and time-of-study group leaders were not explicitly recorded. Therefore, the expenditure of TSh1,942,200 ($242,775) reported by Hall (1977) and mostly financed by the Swedish International Development Authority does not adequately reflect the complete commitment of resources to the "Mtu ni Afya" program. Hall and Dodds (1977) estimated that adding costs of staff time, travel expenses for the 75,000 group leaders, and local distribution costs would increase total campaign costs to TSh4,880,000 ($610,000). Adding an opportunity cost for the time of study, group leaders in training and participation in the programs (at a wage of TSh2 per hour—a low rural wage) would have added TSH4.2 million (525,000), assuming 16 hours for training and 12 hours for participation in the broadcasts. Thus, total project costs would be TSh9,080,-000 ($1,135,000). At this level of expenditure the cost per participant would be TSh4.5 ($0.57) for 2 million participants or TSh7 ($0.87) if one uses an average attendance rate of 65 percent. Costs would also increase substantially if one were to calculate an opportunity cost for the time spent by participants in the program. This opportunity cost would be TSh24 ($3.00) per participant assuming 30 minutes of broadcast and 30 minutes of discussion.

It is necessary to point out that the costs reported above may still be an underestimation of actual costs. For example, the reported costs of producing manuals for 1 million participants was approximately TSh1 ($0.12) for each set of two 48-page booklets. This cost does seem unusually low.

Since the main intention of the campaign was to induce changes in health practices, the cost of these activities must also be assessed. Activities focused on in the campaign included: clearing of standing water, building of latrines, cleansing of drinking water, and wearing of shoes. The main activity that we analyze in terms of disease reduction is the building of latrines. From the data gathered in our sample, we estimated that 980,000 latrines were built. Discussions with villagers led us to estimate that 80 hours of labor were required for building latrines. Hall (1977) reported that 750,000 latrines were built in an estimated 50 hours per latrine. The total labor cost from our estimation would be TSh156.8 million ($19.6 million). Hall's estimation of 50 labor hours per latrine would lead to a somewhat reduced cost. Neither of these estimates includes cost of materials. Assuming that such materials cost the equivalent of two days' wages, the materials cost would be TSh31.4 million ($3.9 million). Gilbert and Jones (1976) reported 16 days of labor and an equivalent cost for materials for a somewhat more elaborate latrine.

Cost-Effectiveness Analysis

There are several potential measures of project effectiveness; these include participation, learning, and changes in health practices. A total registration of 2 million persons was reported. This amount was double the expectations of the project planners. With an estimated attendance rate of 65 percent, we calculate campaign costs on the basis of participants and participant hours as follows:

	Per Registered Participant	Per Attending Participant	Per Registered Participant-Hour	Per Attending Participant-Hour
	(in Tanzanian shillings)			
Externally financed costs	0.97	1.49	0.08	0.12
Plus governmental staff	2.44	3.75	0.20	0.31
Plus group leader time	4.54	7.00	0.38	0.58
Plus participant time	28.54	31.00	2.38	2.58

The registration figure of 2 million represents approximately 25 percent of the adult (over 15 years of age) rural population. Yet our sample of 2,500 revealed a participation rate of 81 percent. This figure may reveal a nonrepresentative sample or misrepresentation of facts or the possibility that many persons in rural areas listened to the programs on an individual rather than group basis and felt that they had participated in the program although records for the campaign would not include them.

On a 25-question test of knowledge regarding health practices, Hall found that those in an experimental group of participants increased test scores from 43 to 63 percent, whereas a control group increased from 49 to 58 percent. The control group increase may represent a weakness in the posttest or a postproject dissemination of knowledge; it may be, too, that some people in the control group actually listened to the program.

Perhaps most important are changes in health practices. Our study of 2,500 people showed that 70 percent saw the need to boil or filter water and 66 percent kept clean water in special containers. Additionally, 58 percent had strong attitudes and 33 percent had moderate attitudes in favor of wearing shoes, whereas 74 percent actually wore shoes. Unfortunately, it is not possible to compare these results with immediate postcampaign health practices, since Hall did not investigate the latter.

Also important is the building and use of latrines. Hall's sample of 2,084 households showed that 939 (45 percent) had latrines after "Mtu ni Afya," whereas only 421 (20 percent) had latrines before the campaign. Our survey of 2,500 persons revealed that 1,475 (59 percent) had constructed latrines after "Mtu ni Afya." Hall's data, extrapolated to the total population, indicate that the immediate result of the campaign was more than doubling of latrines in use. Our data indicate that after four years, latrine usage has increased to include 59 percent of the population. This additional increase may be due to a multiplier effect of persons influencing others, a delayed response to the program, or a normal growth rate, which would have taken place in the absence of the campaign. All three causes probably contributed. Extrapolating the immediate postcampaign increase to the increase over the past few years would show that at least half were directly or indirectly attributable to "Mtu ni Afya." On a cost-effectiveness basis, the campaign investment of TSh40.3 million induced the construction of 980,000 latrines, representing an additional investment of TSh188.2 million.

Cost-Benefit Analysis

The final step in our evaluation of the success of the "Mtu ni Afya" program is an assessment of the benefits derived from changes in health practices. While these changes may include a variety of benefits, we will concentrate upon those that are most easily quantified, particularly changes in disease incidence and subsequent economic benefits of the disease control. These economic benefits take two forms: reduction of treatment costs (a release of medical resources) and an increase in productivity for those no longer suffering from disease.

To estimate the economic benefits from disease reduction, we questioned physicians regarding reduction in disease as a result of "Mtu ni Afya." Primarily for illustrative purposes—and because information was limited—we analyzed a single disease, bilharzia (schistosomiasis). Wen-Pin Chang (1971) reported that schistosomiasis, a parasitic disease, affects 180 million to 200 million people throughout the world. He considered it second only to malaria as a cause of ill health. The World Bank (1975) reported that schistosomiasis is a debilitating disease of varying severity that is transmitted by snails that breed in slow-moving bodies of water. Eliminating standing water, wearing shoes, and using latrines would reduce the impact of schistosomiasis. Therefore, it is necessary to emphasize that the reduction of schistosomiasis requires costs other than those for latrine construction. Hairston (1973) concluded that the use of latrines limited the available breeding grounds for the snails.

While we focus on benefits from reduction of disease, lowered death rates, and shorter periods of illness, other researchers have analyzed the lowered work productivity of those suffering from the disease. For example, Farooq (1964) reviewed four different studies with an average productivity loss of 35 percent. However, Foster

(1967) reported no difference in work productivity for workers on an East African sugarcane estate. MacDonald (1973) reported an average work loss of 14.2 days. We therefore wish to emphasize that the cost-benefit analysis discussed below is an extremely tentative attempt to demonstrate the use of economics for health education decision making. Many of the data are subject to considerable error. However, even if the data used were subject to little error, the technique of cost-benefit analysis should be approached with caution, since many important impacts—for instance, a social policy aimed at improving living conditions without specific productivity changes—are ignored in the quantitative approach.

The effects of latrine usage and the clearing of standing water are clearly reflected in the fact that although the number of latrines in use doubled, the incidence of disease was not reduced proportionately. In fact, as estimated by the physicians we consulted, there was a reduction of only 10 percent. These figures indicate that an individual's health is affected by the health practices of his neighbors. If we had analyzed diseases for which one's health practices had no external effect, we would expect a proportionate reduction. If a disease is carried in unclean water only, and twice as many people drink clean water as a result of a campaign, then the number of people contracting the disease would be halved.

According to physicians' estimates, of the approximately 600,000 people contracting the disease annually, 60,000 fewer persons would contract the disease each year that the latrines built as a result of "Mtu ni Afya" were in use. The incidence of the disease does vary widely in the country. Wright (1973) reported disease incidence ranging as high as 90 percent of the population in some areas. The physicians estimated that 23 percent of the people normally receive treatment at an average cost of TSh70 ($8.75). Therefore, treatment costs as a result of "Mtu ni Afya" are reduced by TSh966,000 ($120,750). Persons who receive treatment remain ill (and are unable to work) for an average of seven days. Assuming 50 working hours (at TSh2 per hour) in the seven days, and assuming that 25 percent of persons with the disease are employed (based on population age distribution), there is an additional work productivity loss of TSh345,000 ($43,125). These figures must be modified slightly by the death rate from the disease. Physicians estimated that 5 percent of those who received treatment would die, whereas the death rate would triple to 15 percent if no treatment were available. The benefits to those who recover from the disease are reduced to TSh327,750 for those who receive treatment. Assuming a cost in productivity of 20 percent for those who do not receive treatment, the benefits are TSh7,854,400. One should note that treatment for schistosomiasis is unpleasant. Davis (1973) reported on the use of several drugs, all with serious side effects—such as vomiting, diarrhea, abdominal pains, weakness, mental illness, anorexia, and jaundice. In an experimental program in Tanzania, he reported that side effects occurred in 50 to 96 percent of those treated. Correlated with the side effects was an increased tendency to discontinue treatment, ranging from 3 to 70 percent. However, the drug with the most side effects was also the most effective, since relapse rates within one year were the lowest when this drug was used.

Assuming that 25 percent of those who contract the disease but recover from it are currently working at minimum rural wages (approximately TSh4,000 per year) and that these individuals would work for an additional 20 years, there would be a total lifetime income cost of TSh80,000. Since this income is received each year and earnings in the future are generally considered less valuable than earnings in the present, it is common practice among economists to use an interest rate and calculate a discounted present value of future income according to the formula:

$$PV = \sum_{i=1}^{n} \frac{W_i}{(1 + r)^i} \qquad (9.1)$$

where W_i is wages in year i (in this case TSh4,000), r is an interest rate (we will use 10 percent), and n is the final year analyzed. The increase in discounted lifetime income will be TSh34,054 ($4,257) for each person who does not contract the disease and die. Therefore, of the 15,000 workers, 3,450 would receive treatment (23 percent) and 173 would die (5 percent). This reduction translates into additional income of TSh5,891,342 ($736,417). For those 11,550 workers who would not receive treatment and for whom the death rate is 15 percent, there would be additional income of TSh58,998,555 ($7,374,819). One should also add future income of those who are not currently in the labor force but will work in the future.

Table 9.3 summarizes the costs for the "Mtu ni Afya" program, building of latrines (costs for shoes and eliminating standing water are ignored), and the subsequent benefits from reduction of incidence of bilharzia. Assuming that all costs are incurred in the first year and that benefits occur in each of the years that latrines are in use, and assuming, in addition, that latrines last only five years and that the interest rate is 10 percent, net benefits are as follows:

$$\text{Net benefits for program} = \sum_{i=1}^{n} \frac{\text{Net benefits in year i}}{(1 + 0.10)^i} \qquad (9.2)$$

$$= \frac{-228.4}{(1.10)} + \frac{74.0}{(1.10)^2} + \frac{74.0}{(1.10)^3} + \frac{74.0}{(1.10)^4} + \frac{74.0}{(1.10)^5} + \frac{74.0}{(1.10)^6}$$

$$= \text{TSh47.48 million (\$5.93 million)}$$

This example, which considers only bilharzia, demonstrates a positive benefit to the program. However, much of the information is estimated. In fact, Hall's estimate on labor cost for latrine building would substantially raise the net benefits to TSh100.20 million ($12.53 million). However, if there is an error in the physicians' estimates, the net benefits could fall dramatically or become negative—for example, if the reduction in disease incidence is only 5 percent, there would be a net loss of TSh81.99 million ($10.25 million). If the interest rate were less than 10 percent, the net benefits would increase, since lower interest rates increase the present value of benefits received in

TABLE 9.3

Summary of Costs and Benefits

Cost	Tanzanian Shillings	U.S. Dollars
"Mtu ni Afya" program		
External	1,942,200	242,775
Tanzanian personnel	2,937,800	367,225
Study group leader time	4,200,000	525,000
Study group, anticipated time	31,200,000	3,900,000
Total (1.3 million attendees)	40,280,000	5,035,000
Latrine building		
Labor	156,800,000	19,600,000
Materials	31,360,000	3,920,000
Total cost (in year 1)	228,440,000	28,555,000
Benefits		
Receive treatment		
Survive	327,750	40,989
Fatal	5,891,342	736,417
Treatment costs	966,000	120,750
No treatment		
Survive	7,854,400	981,800
Fatal	58,998,555	7,374,819
Total benefits (in years 2-6 assuming a five-year life for latrines)	74,038,047	9,254,775

the future. Assuming that the benefits of a 10 percent reduction in disease incidence were realized in a 35 percent increase in work productivity (with no fatalities), the benefits would be only TSh21.96 million per year, yielding a net loss of TSh131.97 million.

Our example, however, was only used to indicate the type of analysis one could use in investigating the costs and benefits of a health education program within the context of conventional economic theory. Even if the benefits had been negative, our example (which only focused on one of the affected diseases) would not necessarily imply the uselessness of the program. The cost-benefit approach relied on changes in work productivity as measured by income only. This is a rather restricted analysis. There are many other more qualitative factors that are as important in judging the benefits of a program. Support for national development, education, and health policies and the potential for improved attitudes are two important positive effects. By concentrating upon income as the main measure of health benefits, cost-benefit analysis may reinforce the cycle of poverty by rejecting investments with costs higher than the income benefits received by low-income workers. The costs are borne by the government through funds received from middle- and higher-income workers and businesses, though their ultimate sources may be different segments of the population. These funds are then distributed to improve education and health conditions for low-income workers, perhaps helping to alleviate poverty in the future. This fund transfer may be more important than the fact that an economic analysis does not reveal sufficient income benefits. In other words, distributional effects may be more important than the magnitude of the benefits.

10
SUMMARY AND CONCLUSIONS

The health problems of developing countries are severe. Infant mortality rates are five to ten times higher than those of developed countries; life spans are 30 to 40 percent lower. The most immediate causes of these poor health statistics are rampant infectious diseases and malnutrition. High disease and malnutrition rates are but two manifestations of the major problem facing developing countries: a low level of economic development. Malnutrition and disease help to ensure the cycle of poverty, since they reduce productivity and earning ability. This lack of income reduces the chances for children to improve their own economic standing. Malnutrition of mothers and infants reduces the intellectual and physical development of the children and places them in a position in which they are less able to succeed at education and at work.

The traditional public health program has directly attacked habits and attitudes that increase the likelihood of disease and malnutrition. Public health programs have also included government measures such as inoculation and elimination of breeding grounds for parasites. The traditional approach to public health falls within the range of a disaggregated policy analysis. Different government agencies deal with different aspects of the poverty problem, with little coordination among them. This lack of coordination among agencies increases the difficulty of solving problems. The difficulty is not that agencies work at cross purposes, since one would expect a general consistency among a given society's institutions in terms of economic relationships and cultural values. Rather, the difficulty is that no single agency is equipped to question the economic relationships and cultural values in which its own decisions are made. These difficulties are further compounded by an international economic structure that tends to be dominated by multinational corporations and limits the economic independence of developing countries.

If inoculations exist as a preventive measure for disease, it is reasonable to expect that these measures will be adopted and reduce disease. To the extent that disease results from unsanitary conditions connected with poverty, the probable success of disease eradication programs is reduced. Malnutrition is partially a function of ignorance, but it is mostly a consequence of lack of food or of purchasing ability. Lack of food is related to a nation's agricultural policies. These policies often result in centralized control of single-, cash-crop plantations. Much arable land is used to grow coffee, cocoa, sugar, tobacco, and flowers to meet the demands of a domestic elite and of multinational corporations. Many studies of agriculture have shown that the small farm tends to be more efficient than the large farm. The appropriate public health programs may be land redistribution and conversion of this land, where possible, to multiple-, nutritious-crop agriculture.

Lack of purchasing power can only be eliminated for the long term by creating a stable economic base. Urban poverty areas are growing in size as many countries experience a massive rural-to-urban migration owing to the lack of economic opportunities in rural areas. The appropriate public health program for this cause of malnutrition seems to be a diversion of resources to rural areas to develop the economic base there. These resources include some degree of decentralized industrialization and a redistribution of landownership with resources available to support the prosperity of smaller farms.

These public health programs focus more on economic structure than have traditional programs. Changes in economic structure require major changes in the social structure and power relationships that exist in a society, whether the change is to socialism or decentralized capitalism. Without such changes, traditional programs to reduce disease and malnutrition are not likely to be successful.

BIBLIOGRAPHY

Abell, H. C. 1968. Farm Radio Forum Project: Ghana 1964-65. Paris: United Nations Educational, Scientific and Cultural Organization.

Apted, F. I. G., W. E. Ornerod, D. P. Smyly, B. W. Stronbach, and E. L. Szlamp. 1963. "A Comparative Study of the Epidemiology of Endemic Rhodesian Sleeping Sickness in Different Parts of Africa." Journal of Tropical Medicine and Hygiene 66: 1-16.

Arrow, K. J. 1973. "Higher Education as a Filter." Journal of Public Economics 2: 193-216.

Ashby, J., S. Klees, D. Pachico, and S. Wells. 1978. The Economics of Education and Communications System Strategies for Agricultural Development. Washington, D.C.: Agency for International Development.

Barlow, R. 1967. "Economic Effects of Malaria Eradication." American Economic Review 57: 139-57.

Barnet, R., and R. Muller. 1974a. "A Reporter at Large: The Multinational Corporations." New Yorker, December 2, pp. 53-56.

_____. 1974b. Global Reach. New York: Simon and Schuster.

Basta, S. S., and A. Churchill. 1974. Iron Deficiency Anemia and the Productivity of Adult Males in Indonesia. Staff Working Paper no. 175. Washington, D.C.: International Bank for Reconstruction and Development.

Bates, D., and G. Donaldson. 1975. "Changes in Emphasis in Rural Sector Lending." Finance and Development 12: 23-27.

Becker, G. S. 1964. Human Capital. New York: National Bureau of Economic Research.

_____. 1965. "A Theory of the Allocation of Time." Economic Journal 75: 493-517.

Belli, P. 1971. "The Economic Implications of Malnutrition: The Dismal Science Revisited." Economic Development and Cultural Change 20: 1-23.

Bengoa, J. M. 1970. Curative Aspects of Malnutrition and Rehabilitation of the Malnourished Child. Eastern Mediterranean Region Food and Nutrition Seminar. Beirut: United Nations International Children's Emergency Fund.

Berg, A. 1973. The Nutrition Factor: Its Role in National Development. Washington, D.C.: Brookings Institution.

Berg, A., and R. Muscat. 1973. "Nutrition Program Planning: An Approach." In Nutrition, National Development and Planning, edited by A. Berg, N. Scrimshaw, and D. Call, pp. 247-74. Cambridge: Massachusetts Institute of Technology Press.

Blanca, T. A., and G. C. Graham. 1974. "The High Cost of Being Poor: Water." Archives of Environmental Health 28: 312-15.

Blaug, M., P. R. G. Layard, and M. Woodhall. 1969. The Causes of Graduate Unemployment in India. London: Penguin Press.

Bodenheimer, T. S. 1969. "Mobile Units: A Solution to the Rural Health Problem." Medical Care 7: 144-54.

Borgstrom, G. 1974. The Food and People Dilemma. Cambridge, Mass.: Duxbury Press.

Bowles, S., and H. Gintis. 1973. "IQ in the U.S. Class Structure." Social Policy 3: 65-96.

Brown, L., and E. Eckholm. 1974. By Bread Alone. New York: Praeger.

Bryant, J. 1969. Health and the Developing World. Ithaca, N.Y.: Cornell University Press.

Buchanan, R. 1975. "Breast-Feeding: Aid to Infant Health and Fertility Control." Population Reports 8: 54-55.

Burk, M. C., and M. Ezekiel. 1967. "Food and Nutrition in Developing Countries." In Agricultural Development and Economic Growth, edited by H. Southworth and B. Johnston. Ithaca, N.Y.: Cornell University Press.

Caldwell, H. R., and D. W. Dunlop. 1977. "An Empirical Study of Health Planning in Latin America and Africa." Presented at the American Public Health Association Meeting, Washington, D.C., November.

Cesario, F. J., S. R. Simon, and I. L. Kinne. 1970. The Economics of Malnutrition. Columbus, Ohio: Battelle Memorial Institute.

Chapra, Gomacho, Devany, and Thomson. 1970. "Maternal Nutrition and Family Planning." American Journal of Clinical Nutrition 23: 1043-58.

Chernichovsky, D. 1977. "Household Economics and Impact Measurement of Nutrition and Health Related Programs. Presented at the Pan American Health Organization Conference on Impact Measurement, Panama, August.

Childers, V. E. 1969. "Infant Nutrition: Priority for Development." International Development Review 13: 13-15.

Chossey, J. P., A. G. Van Veen, and F. W. Young. 1967. "The Application of Social Science Research Methods to the Study of Food Habits and Food Consumption in an Industrializing Area." American Journal of Clinical Nutrition 29: 56-64.

Clearinghouse on Development Communication: The Pila Project— Guatemala. 1977. Washington, D.C.: Academy for Educational Development.

Clower, R., et al. 1976. Growth without Development: An Economic Survey of Liberia. Evanston, Ill.: Northwestern University Press.

Cochrane, A. L. 1972. "Effectiveness and Efficiency." In Random Reflections on Health Services. London: Nuffeld Provincial Hospitals Trust.

Cohen, H. A. 1967. "Variations in Cost among Hospitals of Different Sizes." Southern Economic Journal 33: 355-66.

Cohn, E. 1976. The Economics of Education. Cambridge, Mass.: Ballinger.

Colle, R. 1977. "Guatemala: The Traditional Laundering Place as a Nonformal Health Education Setting." Convergence 10: 32-39.

Cooke, T. M., and S. T. Romweber. 1977. "Radio Nutrition Education—A Test of the Advertising Technique: Philippines and Nicaragua." Unpublished. Manoff International, Washington, D.C.

Correa, H. 1968. "Nutrition, Working Capacity, Productivity, and Economic Growth." Presented at the Western Hemisphere Nutrition Congress II, San Juan, Puerto Rico, August.

Correa, H., and G. Cummins. 1970. "Contribution of Nutrition to Economic Growth." American Journal of Clinical Nutrition 23: 560–65.

Cosminsky, S. 1977. "The Role and Training of Traditional Midwives: Policy Implications for Maternal and Child Health Care." Presented at the Latin American and African Studies Associations Meeting, Houston, November.

Coursin, D. B. 1963. "Undernutrition and Brain Function." Borden's Review of Nutrition Research 26: 1–16.

Cravioto, J. 1966. "Malnutrition and Behavioral Development in the Preschool Child." In Preschool Child Malnutrition: Primary Deterrent to Human Progress. Washington, D.C.: National Academy of Sciences.

Cravioto, J., and E. R. DeLicardie. 1968. "Intersensory Development of School Age Children." In Malnutrition, Learning, and Behavior, edited by N. Scrimshaw and J. E. Gordon. Boston, Mass.: Massachusetts Institute of Technology Press.

Cravioto, J., L. Hambraeus, and B. Vahlquist. 1974. Early Malnutrition and Mental Development. Uppsala: Swedish Nutrition Foundation.

Cravioto, J., and B. Robles. 1965. "Evolution of Adaptive and Motor Behavior during Rehabilitation from Kwashiorkor." American Journal of Orthopsychiatry 35: 449–64.

Crystal, R. A., and A. Brewster. 1966. "Cost-Benefit and Cost-Effectiveness in the Health Field." Inquiry 3: 1–14.

Cuca, R., and C. S. Pierce. 1978. Experiments in Family Planning: Lessons from the Developing World. Washington, D.C.: World Bank.

David, A. S., and A. R. Omran. 1974. "Economies and Community Medicine." Community Medicine in Developing Countries, edited by A. R. Omran. New York: Springer.

Davis, A. 1973. "Chemotherapy in Control." In Epidemiology and Control of Schistosomiasis, edited by N. Ansari. Baltimore: University Park Press.

Dayton, D. H. 1969. "Early Malnutrition and Human Development." Children 16: 211-17.

De La Rue, A. 1967. "Ujamaa on the March." New African 6 (October): 10.

Denison, E. F. 1962. The Source of Economic Growth in the United States. Washington, D.C.: Committee for Economic Development.

Dighe, A., and P. Roy. 1977. Factors Affecting Comprehension and Retention of Selected S.I.T.E. Programs. New Delhi: Council for Social Development.

Djukanovic, V., and E. P. Mach, eds. 1975. Alternative Approaches to Meeting Basic Health Needs in Developing Countries. Geneva: World Health Organization.

Duckham, A. N., J. G. W. Jones, and E. H. Roberts, eds. 1976. Food Production and Consumption. New York: Elsevier.

El-Nazar, H. 1958. "Control of Schistosomiasis in the Gegvia, Sudan." Journal of Tropical Pediatrics 14: 55-58.

Eyer, J., and P. Sterling. 1977. "Stress-Related Mortality and Social Organization." Review of Radical Political Economics 9: 1-44.

Farooq, M. 1964. "Medical and Economic Importance of Schistosomiasis." Journal of Tropical Medicine and Hygiene 67: 105-12.

Feldstein, M. S. 1964. "Net Social Benefit Calculation and the Public Investment Decision." Oxford Economic Papers 5: 114-31.

Florencis, C., and R. E. Evenson. N.d. "Economic, Demographic, Health, and Nutritional Factors in Rural Household Behavior." Unpublished.

Forbes, W. H. 1967. "Longevity and Medical Costs." New England Journal of Medicine 277: 71-78.

Foster, R. 1967. "Schistosomiasis on an Irrigated Estate in East Africa." Journal of Tropical Medicine and Hygiene 70: 133-40, 185-95.

Fougeyrollas, P. 1967. Television and the Social Education of Women—A First Report on the UNESCO-Senegal Pilot Project at Dakar. Reports and Papers in Mass Communication no. 50. Paris: United Nations Educational, Scientific and Cultural Organization.

Fuchs, V. R. 1972. Essays in the Economics of Health and Medical Care. New York: National Bureau of Economic Research.

_____. 1974. "Some Economic Aspects of Mortality in Developed Countries." In The Economics of Health and Medical Care, edited by M. Perlman. New York: Macmillan.

Galbraith, J. K. 1967. The New Industrial State. New York: Signet.

Gilbert, G., and W. I. Jones. 1976. PNP VII Rubber Estate Anemia Case. Washington, D.C.: World Bank.

Gintis, H. 1971. "Education Technology and the Characteristics of Worker Productivity." American Economic Review 61: 266-79.

Gish, O. 1970. "Health Planning in Developing Countries." Journal of Development Studies 6: 67-76.

_____. 1973. "Resource Allocation, Equality of Access, and Health." International Journal of Health Services 3: 399-412.

Gopalan, C. 1958. "Studies on Lactation in Poor Indian Communities." Journal of Tropical Pediatrics 4: 87-97.

Gordon, J. E. 1969. "Nutrition Science and Society." Nutrition Reviews 27: 331-38.

Green, L. W. 1974. "Toward Cost-Benefit Evaluations of Health Education: Some Concepts, Methods, and Examples." Health Education Monographs 2: 36-64.

_____. 1977a. "Utilization of Cost-Effectiveness in Evaluation in the Health Care Field." In Health Care and Evaluation Research, edited by L. Bowman, T. J. Northcutt, Jr., and E. C. Main. University of South Florida.

_____. 1977b. "Evaluation and Measurement: Some Dilemmas for Health Education." American Journal of Public Health 67: 155-61.

Grossman, M. 1972. The Demand for Health: A Theoretical and Empirical Investigation. New York: Columbia University Press.

Gueri, M. 1975. Evaluation of a Breast-Feeding Campaign in Trinidad. Kingston: Caribbean Food and Nutrition Institute.

Guttmacher, S., and R. Danielson. 1977. "Changes in Urban Health Care: An Argument against Technological Pessimism." International Journal of Health Services 7: 383-400.

Guzman, M. 1968. "Impaired Physical Growth and Malnutrition in Malnourished Populations." In Malnutrition, Learning, and Behavior, edited by N. Scrimshaw and J. W. Gordon, pp. 42-54. Cambridge: Massachusetts Institute of Technology Press.

Hairston, N. G. 1973. "The Dynamics of Transmission." In Epidemiology and Control of Schistosomiasis, edited by N. Ansari. Baltimore: University Park Press.

Hakim, P., and G. Solimano. 1975. Nutrition and National Development: Establishing the Connection. Institute of Nutrition Planning, Discussion Paper no. 5. Cambridge, Mass.: Massachusetts Institute of Technology Press.

Hall, B. L. 1975. Adult Education and the Development of Socialism in Tanzania. Dar es Salaam: East African Publishing Bureau.

_____. 1977. "Tanzania's Health Campaign: Mtu ni Afya." Unpublished. Swedish International Development Authority, Institute of Development Studies, University of Sussex, and International Council for Adult Education, Ottawa.

Hall, B. L., and T. Dodds. 1977. "Voices for Development: The Tanzanian National Radio Study Campaigns." In Radio for Education and Development: Case Studies, edited by P. L. Spain, D. T. Jamison, and E. G. McAnany. Washington, D.C.: World Bank.

Hall, T. 1974. "Estimating Requirements and Supply: Where Do We Stand?" In Pan American Conference on Health Manpower Planning. Washington, D.C.: Pan American Health Organization.

Harris, M. 1975. "The Kenya Radio Series Which Teaches as It Entertains, and How You Can Do It." Unpublished memorandum. Nairobi: United Nations Educational, Scientific and Cultural Organization.

Harrison, G. G. 1978. "Strategies for Solving World Food Problems." In Nutrition in Economic and Social Development, edited by P. Pearson. Tucson: University of Arizona Press.

Heller, P. S. 1973. "The Strategy of Health-Sector Planning." In Public Health in the People's Republic of China, edited by Myron E. Wegman et al. New York: Josiah Macy, Jr., Foundation.

Higgins, M., and J. Montague. 1972. "Nutrition Education through the Mass Media in Korea." Journal of Nutrition Education 4: 58-62.

Hollant, E. 1977. Radio Docteur—Health Education Radio Program of the Centre d'Hygiene Familiale. Port-au-Prince: Centre d'Hygiene Familiale.

Hostetler, S. 1976. Health Messages through Humor. ICIT Report no. 15. Washington, D.C.: Agency for International Development.

Hughes, C., and J. Hunter. 1970. "Disease and Development in Africa." Social Science and Medicine 3: 443-93.

Hunter, J. M. 1966. "River Blindness in Nanzodi, Northern Ghana: A Hypothesis of Cyclical Advance and Retreat." Geographical Review 56: 398-416.

Institute of Adult Education. 1974. "Mtu ni Afya: An Evaluation of the 1973 Mass Health Education Campaign in Tanzania." Studies in Adult Education, no. 12. Dar es Salaam: Institute of Adult Education, June.

Jamison, D., S. Klees, and S. Wells. 1978. The Costs of Educational Media: Guidelines for Planning and Evaluation. Beverly Hills, Calif.: Sage.

Jamison, D., P. Suppes, and S. Wells. 1974. "The Effectiveness of Alternative Instructional Media: A Survey." Review of Educational Research 44: 1-67.

Jay, L. 1973. "Food and Nutrition Planning." Journal of Agricultural Economics, vol. 14.

Jelliffe, D. B. 1966. The Assessment of the Nutritional Status of the Community: With Special Reference to Field Surveys in Developing Regions of the World. World Health Organization Research Monograph no. 66. Geneva.

Jelliffe, D. B., and P. E. F. Jelliffe. 1975. "Human Milk, Nutrition and the World Resource Crises." Science 188: 557-61.

_____. 1977. "The Infant Food Industry and International Child Health." International Journal of Health Services 7: 249-54.

Jensen, A. 1969. "How Much Can We Boast IQ and Scholastic Achievement." Harvard Education Review 39: 1-123.

Johnston, B. F., and J. W. Millar. 1960. "The Nature of Agriculture's Contribution to Economic Development." Food Research Institute Studies, vol. 1.

Jordan, J. L. 1977. "Improved Health and Increased Productivity in Low-Income Nations: The Integrated Delivery of Rural Health Care." Presented at the Latin American and African Studies Associations Meeting, Houston, November.

Kallen, D. J. 1969. "Nutrition and Society." Paper presented at the Conference on Nutrition and Human Development, Michigan State University, East Lansing, May.

Kamarck, A. M. 1976. The Tropics and Economic Development: A Provocative Inquiry into the Poverty of Nations. Washington, D.C.: World Bank.

Klarman, H. E., J. O. Francis, and G. D. Rosenthal. 1968. "Cost Effectiveness Analysis Applied to the Treatment of Chronic Renal Disease." Medical Care 6: 48-54.

Klees, S., and S. Wells. 1977. Cost-Effectiveness and Cost-Benefit Analysis for Educational Planning and Evaluation: Methodology and Application to Instructional Technology. Washington, D.C.: Agency for International Development.

_____. 1978. Cost Analysis for Education Decision Making. Washington, D.C.: Agency for International Development.

Kleiman, F. 1974. "The Determinants of National Outlay on Health." In The Economics of Health and Medical Care, edited by M. Perlman. New York: Macmillan.

Kleinbach, J. 1974. "Social Structure and the Education of Health Personnel." International Journal of Health Services 4: 297-317.

Kraut, H. A., and E. A. Muller. 1946. "Calorie Intake and Industrial Output." Science 104: 495-97.

Kreimer, O. (Rapporteur). 1977. International Conference on Nutrition Education, Manila, April.

Krishnamurthy, L. 1976. "Nutrition Education—The Indian Case." In Nutrition Planning in the Developing World, edited by M. A. Anderson and T. Grewal. New York: CARE.

Kugelmoss, N. L., L. E. Poull, and E. L. Samuel. 1964. "Nutritional Improvement of Child Mentality." American Journal of the Medical Sciences 218: 631-33.

Lanoix, J. N. 1958. "Relation between Engineering and Bilharzia." Bulletin of the World Health Organization 18: 1011.

Lappé, F. M. 1975a. "The Banality of Hunger." In Food for People —Not for Profit, edited by C. Lerga and M. Jacobson. New York: Ballantine.

_____. 1975b. Diet for a Small Planet. New York: Ballantine.

Lappé, F. M., and J. Collins. 1977. Food First: Beyond the Myth of Scarcity. Boston: Houghton Mifflin.

Lele, U. 1975. The Design of Rural Development: Lessons from Africa. Baltimore: Johns Hopkins University Press.

Leslie, J. 1978a. "The Use of Health Statistics as an Effectiveness Measure in Certain Development Communications Projects." In Economics of Educational Technology, vol. 2. Paris: United Nations Educational, Scientific and Cultural Organization.

_____. 1978b. "The Use of Mass Media in Health Education Campaigns." Educational Broadcasting International 11: 136-42.

"Lesotho Distance Teaching Centre: An Experiment with Educational Radio Spots." 1976. Maseru, Lesotho, January 1976.

Lloyd-Still, J. D. 1976. Malnutrition and Intellectual Development. Lancaster, England: MTP Press.

MacDonald, G. 1973. "Measurement of the Clinical Manifestations of Schistosomiasis." In Epidemiology and Control of Schistosomiasis, edited by N. Ansari. Baltimore: University Park Press.

Mahai, B. A. P., et al. 1975. "The Second Follow-up Formative Evaluation Report of the 'Food Is Life' Campaign." Dar es Salaam: Institute of Adult Education.

Malenbaum, W. 1970. "Health and Productivity in Poor Areas." In Empirical Studies in Health Economics, edited by H. Klarman. Baltimore: Johns Hopkins University Press.

_____. 1973. "Health and Expansion in Poor Lands." International Journal of Health Services 3: 161-76.

Maliyamkono, T. L. 1977. "Educational Reforms for Development: A Review of the Tanzanian Approach." Unpublished manuscript. Washington, D.C.: World Bank.

Manoff International. 1976. Changing Nutrition and Health Behavior through the Mass Media: Nicaragua and the Philippines. New York: Manoff International.

Marglin, S. A. 1967. Public Investment Criteria: Benefit-Cost Analysis for Planned Economic Growth. Cambridge, Mass.: Harvard University Press.

Mathur, J., and P. Neurath. 1959. An Indian Experiment in Farm Radio Forums. Paris: United Nations Educational, Scientific and Cultural Organization.

Matiko, J. M. M. 1976. "Radio Campaigns for Adult Education in Tanzania." Presented to the International Conference on Communication Policy and Planning for Education and Development, Stanford University, July 15.

May, J. M., and H. Lemons. 1969. "The Ecology of Malnutrition." Journal of the American Medical Association 207: 2401-5.

McKigney, J. I. 1968. "Economic Aspects of Infant Feeding Practices in the West Indies." Journal of Tropical Pediatrics 14: 55-58.

Mellor, J. W., and U. J. Lele. 1972. "Growth Linkages of the New Foodgrain Production Technologies." Occasional Paper no. 50, Cornell University, Ithaca, N.Y.

Monckeberg, R. 1968. "Effect of Early Marasmic Malnutrition of Subsequent Physical and Psychological Development." In Malnutrition, Learning, and Behavior, edited by N. Scrimshaw and J. E. Gordon. Boston, Mass.: Massachusetts Institute of Technology Press.

Mushkin, S. 1962. "Health as an Investment." Journal of Political Economy 70: 129-57.

Myrdal, G. 1968. Asian Drama: An Inquiry into the Poverty of Nations. New York: Pantheon.

Nader, R., M. Green, and J. Seligman. 1976. Taming the Giant Corporation. New York: W. W. Norton.

Nash, H. 1974. "Life Blooms in the Rapti Valley." War on Hunger: A Report from A.I.D. 8: 11-15.

Navarro, V. 1975. "The Political Economy of Medical Care." International Journal of Health Services 5: 65-94.

_____. 1977. "Political Power, the State, and Their Implications in Medicine." Review of Radical Political Economics 9: 61-80.

Newell, K. 1975. Health by the People. Geneva: World Health Organization.

Nicol, J., et al. 1954. Canada's Farm Radio Forum. Paris: United Nations Educational, Scientific and Cultural Organization.

North, A. F., Jr. 1970. "Research Issues in Child Health: A Head-start Research Seminar." Pediatrics 45: 669-701.

Oettinger, A. G., and N. Zapol. 1972. "Will Information Technologies Help Learning?" Teachers College Record 74: 3-54.

Oshima, H. T. 1967. "Food Consumption, Nutrition, and Economic Development in Asian Countries." Economic Development and Cultural Change 15: 385-97.

PAG Secretariat. 1976. "A Pilot Study of the Feasibility of Using Mass Media for Importing Nutrition Education in Haharashtra, India —Part VI Case Histories in Mass Communication." PAG Bulletin, vol. 6 (March).

Parlato, R. 1974. "Advertising and Mass Communications: A Model for Rural Nutrition Information Programs." PAG Bulletin 4: 17-18.

Patton, D. 1968. The United States and World Resources. New York: Van Nostrand.

Puffer, R., and C. Serrano. 1971. Patterns of Mortality in Child-hood. Washington, D.C.: Pan American Health Organization.

Rawls, J. 1971. A Theory of Justice. Cambridge, Mass.: Harvard University Press.

Reutlinger, S., and M. Selowsky. 1976. Malnutrition and Poverty: Magnitude and Policy Options. Washington, D.C.: World Bank.

Revelle, R. 1974. "Food and Population." Scientific American 231: 160-70.

Rice, D. P. 1966. Estimating the Cost of Illness. Washington, D.C.: U.S. Department of Health, Education and Welfare.

Rodberg, L., and G. Stevenson. 1977. "The Health Care Industry in Advanced Capitalism." Review of Radical Political Economics 9: 104-15.

Rody, N. 1978. "Things Go Better with Coconuts—Program Strategies in Micronesia." Journal of Nutrition Education 10: 19-22.

Roemer, M. 1977. Health Income Distribution and Source of Health Expenditures in Developing Countries. Los Angeles: University of California.

Rogers, E., and F. Shoemaker. 1971. Communication of Innovation. New York: Free Press.

Rosenthal, G. D. 1974. "The Demand for General Hospital Facilities." Hospital Monograph Series no. 14, American Medical Association, Chicago.

Ruchlin, H. S., and D. C. Rogers. 1973. Economics and Health Care. Springfield, Ill.: Thomas.

Sagan, C. 1977. Dragons of Eden: Speculations on the Evolution of Human Intelligence. New York: Random House.

Schramm, W. 1977. Big Media, Little Media. Beverly Hills, Calif.: Sage.

Schuftan, C. 1977. "The Challenge of Feeding the People: Chile under Allende and Tanzania under Nyerere." Latin American Studies Association and African Studies Association Annual Meetings, Houston, November.

_____. 1978. "Nutrition Planning—What Relevance to Hunger?" Food Policy 3: 59-65.

_____. N.d. "Household Purchasing Power Deficit: A More Operational Indicator to Express Malnutrition. Unpublished.

Schuftan, C., N. Ozerol, and J. Carter. 1977. Nutrition Planning Model. Nashville, Tenn.: MCH/FP Center, Meharry Medical College.

Schultz, T. W. 1960. "Capital Formation by Education." Journal of Political Economy 68: 571-83.

_____. 1961. "Investment in Human Capital." American Economic Review 51: 1-17.

_____. 1963. The Economic Value of Education. New York: Columbia University Press.

Schumacher, E. F. 1973. Small Is Beautiful. New York: New Library.

Scott, D. 1957. "The Epidemiology of Human Trypanosomiasis in Ashanti, Ghana." Journal of Tropical Medicine and Hygiene 60: 205-14, 238-49, 257-74, 302-15.

Scrimshaw, N. S. 1967. "Malnutrition, Learning and Behavior."
American Journal of Clinical Nutrition 20: 493-502

_____. 1974. "Nutrition and Infection." In Recent Advances in Hu-
man Nutrition, edited by J. Brock. London.

Scrimshaw, N. S., C. E. Taylor, and J. E. Gordon. 1968. Inter-
actions of Nutrition and Infection. Geneva: World Health Organization.

Segall, M. 1972. "The Politics of Health in Tanzania." Development and Change, vol. 4, no. 1. London and Beverly Hills:
Sage.

Seidel, V. 1972. "The Barefoot Doctor in the People's Republic of
China." New England Journal of Medicine 286: 1292-1300.

Selowsky, M. 1971. "An Attempt to Estimate Rates of Return to Investment in Human Energy." Presented at the International Conference on Nutrition, National Development, and Planning, Massachusetts Institute of Technology.

_____. 1973. "A Note on Pre-School Age Investment in Human Capi-
tal in Developing Countries." Presented at the Workshop on
Economics of Education, World Bank, Washington, D.C., October.

Selowsky, M., and L. Taylor. 1971. "The Economics of Malnourished Children: A Study of Disinvestment in Human Capital."
Discussion Paper no. 13, Center for Economic Research, University of Minnesota.

Shivji, I. G. 1975. Class Struggles in Tanzania. Dar es Salaam:
Tanzania.

Smith, H. J. 1974. "Barefoot Doctors and the Medical Pyramid."
British Medical Journal 2: 429-32.

Smith, W. 1968. "Cost-Effectiveness and Cost-Benefit Analyses for
Public Health Programs." Public Health Reports 83: 899-906.

Sorkin, A. 1974. "Education and Income in Chile." Journal of Economic Studies, vol. 1.

_____. 1976. Health Economics in Developing Countries. Lexington,
Mass.: D. C. Heath.

Spence, M. A. 1973. Market Signalling. Cambridge, Mass.: Harvard University Press.

Stine, O. C., J. B. Saratsiotis, and O. F. Furno. 1967. "Appraising the Health of Culturally Deprived Children." American Journal of Clinical Nutrition 20: 1084-95.

Stoch, M. B., and P. M. Smythe. 1967. "The Effect of Undernutrition during Infancy on Subsequent Brain Growth and Intellectual Development." South African Medical Journal, vol. 41.

_____. 1968. "Undernutrition during Infancy and Subsequent Brain Growth and Intellectual Development." In Malnutrition, Learning, and Behavior, edited by N. Scrimshaw and J. E. Gordon. Boston: Massachusetts Institute of Technology Press.

Thompson, A. A. 1975. "Corporate Bigness—For Better or for Worse?" Sloan Management Review 17: 37-60.

Tudge, C. 1977. The Famine Business. London: St. Martin's Press.

Turnham, D. 1971. The Employment Problem in Less Developed Countries. Paris: Organization for Economic Cooperation and Development.

Udry, J. R., et al. 1972. "Can Mass Media Advertising Increase Contraceptive Use?" Family Planning Perspectives 4: 37-44.

Van Etten, G. 1972. "Toward Research on Health Development in Tanzania." Social Science and Medicine 6: 335-52.

Waddy, B. B. 1966. "Medical Problems Arising from the Lakes in Tropical Africa." In Man Made Lakes, edited by L. McConnell. London: Academic Press.

Wai, V. T. 1975. "Some Economic Concepts and Policy Issues in Developing Countries." Finance and Development 12: 27-31.

Weisbrod, B. 1961. Economics of Public Health. Philadelphia: University of Pennsylvania Press.

Weisbrod, B. A. 1962. "Education and Investment in Human Capital." Journal of Political Economy 70: 106-23.

_____. 1971. "Costs and Benefits of Medical Research: A Case Study of Poliomyelitis." Journal of Political Economy 79: 527-42.

Wells, S. 1976. Instructional Technology in Developing Countries: Decision Making Processes in Education. New York: Praeger.

Wen-Pin Chang. 1971. "Major Health Problems in the Practice of Medicine in Developing Countries." Ethiopian Medical Journal 9: 161-77.

Winick, M., and P. Rosso. 1969. "The Effect of Severe Early Malnutrition on Cellular Growth of Human Brain." Pediatric Research 3: 181-84.

Winslow, C. 1951. The Cost of Sickness and the Price of Health. Geneva: World Health Organization.

Woodruff, C. W. 1966. "An Analysis of the I.C.N.N.D. Data on Physical Growth of the Pre-School Child. In Pre-School Child Malnutrition: Primary Deterrent to Human Progress. Washington, D.C.: National Academy of Sciences.

World Bank. 1975. Health Sector Policy Paper. Baltimore: Johns Hopkins University Press.

Wright, W. H. 1973. "Geographical Distribution of Schistosomes and Their Intermediate Hosts." In Epidemiology and Control of Schistosomiasis, edited by N. Ansari. Baltimore: University Park Press.

Zeitlan, M. F., and C. Formacion. 1977. "The HIID/U.P. College Iloilo Evaluation of the Manoff International Nutrition Education Radio Advertising Campaign in Iloilo, Philippines: October 1975-October 1976." Unpublished. Harvard Institute for International Development, Cambridge, Mass.

Zukin, P. 1975. "Health and Economic Development: How Significant Is the Relationship?" International Development Review 17: 17-21.

INDEX

Abell, H. C. , 114
Adult Education Year, 106
advertising: of birth control, 99;
  and breast feeding, 86 (see also
  mass media)
American Medical Association, 65
anemia, 68
annualization factor, 53
anorexia, 133
anthropometry in health status, 58
Apted, F. I. G. , 83
Arrow, K. J. , 70
Arusha Declaration of 1967, 107,
  108, 109, 111
Ashby, J. , 29

backslider effect, 99
Bangladesh: facility access in, 38;
  health care strategies in, 22;
  rice yields in, 41
Barlow, R. , 82
Barnet, R. , 41, 42
Basta, S. S. , 68, 96
Bates, D. , 29
Becker, G. S. , 50, 70
beef consumption, 40
Belli, P. , 14
Berg, A. , 26, 39, 71, 83, 100
bilharzia (schistosomiasis), 12,
  68, 121, 122, 123, 131, 133-35
biochemical test analysis in health
  status, 58
birth control: advertising of, 99;
  incentives for, 59; and mass
  media, 94
birth weight and nutrition, 33
birthrates: in developing countries, 5, 33; and population control, 82
Blanca, T. A. , 12, 33

Blaug, M. , 71
blindness, disease-related, 12
Bodenheimer, T. S. , 56
Bolivia, health care spending
  in, 5
Borgstrom, G. , 39, 40
Bowles, S. , 30, 70
brain development: and intelligence, 13; and malnutrition,
  13-14
Brazil: crops in, 41; health
  care spending in, 5
bread, white, 42
breast feeding: and advertising,
  86; and economic problems, 82-
  83; and education, 90
Brewster, A. , 43
Brown, L. , 40, 41
Buchanan, R. , 83

Caldwell, H. R. , 9, 12, 34, 38
caloric intake: in developed/de-
  veloping countries, 79-80; and
  regression analysis, 101; and
  worker productivity, 67 (see
  also food consumption, nutrition)
Canada, media in, 114
capital formation and population,
  80
capitalism: decentralized, 138;
  investment capital requirements
  of, 31
carbohydrates, production of, 40
Carter, J. , 26, 28
cash crops, 41
Cesario, F. J. , 43, 67, 71, 75,
  95, 99
Ceylon, mortality rates in, 82
"Chakula ni Uhai, " 115
Chapra, 14

157